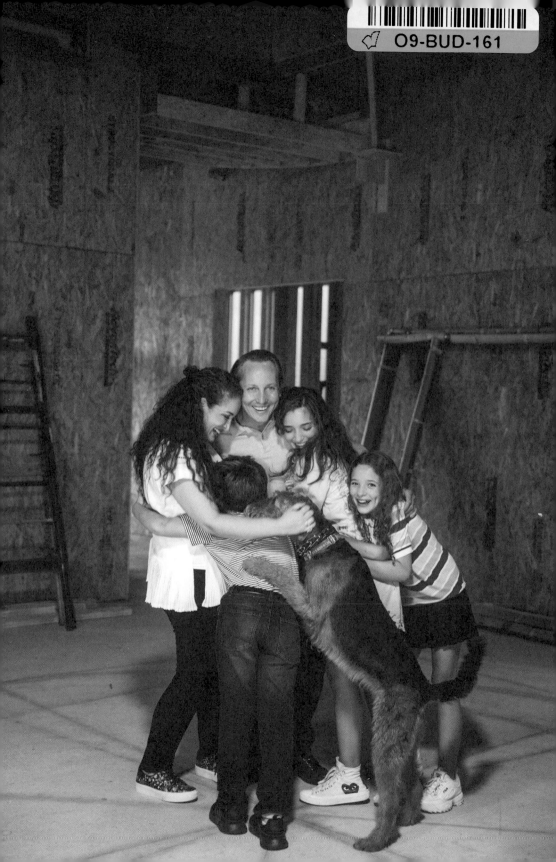

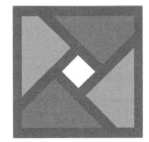

CUCO PRESS

Continue the journey by following my podcast, *On My Way*.
Subscribe wherever you get your podcasts.

You can also find more at LorenaJuncoMargain.com or
Instagram (@Lorenajuncomargain), Twitter (@ljuncomargain),
Facebook, and YouTube.

PRAISE FOR *ON THE WAY TO CASA LOTUS*

I've seen firsthand my friend Lorena's choice to come out of the darkness and into the light and to find forgiveness instead of grieve. Her journey is one we can all learn from and find inspiration in.

—**Camila Alves McConaughey, entrepreneur, philanthropist, founder of WomenOfToday.com**

In this beautifully written book, Lorena Junco Margain brings immense insight into teaching us about the practice of the injured becoming the healer. Her remarkable grace and ability to forgive expands bonds and breaks barriers. *On the Way to Casa Lotus* is a poignant reminder that people make mistakes, and that when we do, we must start again and try to do better. Surgeons like myself are reminded of our limitations as humans and our vocation to cure when able, but to heal always.

—**Nancy D. Perrier, MD, FACS, chief of surgical endocrinology, University of Texas MD Anderson Cancer Center**

Unapologetically bold in its expression of vulnerability and pain, this exquisite narrative invites readers deep into the mind and heart of a woman wronged yet determined to make things right—not merely for herself, but for the world. Steeped in the redeeming love of Junco Margain's close-knit Mexican family—who have preserved their unity and cultural heritage despite their own profound traumas—*On the Way to Casa Lotus* bravely and poetically redefines the boundaries between the personal and the universal. A beacon of hope for women everywhere, it invites all those struggling in silence to let their voices be heard.

—**Reem Acra, designer, Reem Acra New York**

On the Way to Casa Lotus is a book about hope. The author's journey to transforming the violent acts of surgery and a surgeon's grave mistake into a quest for physical and spiritual balance holds much wisdom about how to be proactive and creative in the face of illness. It is a poignant reminder to readers and the medical community that illness affects not only the afflicted but also their family and loved ones; that bodies are not a set of separate parts, but rather are whole—and one with the soul. This book is an invitation to all to create our own rituals, follow our intuitions, and allow pain to help us grow.

—**Prune Nourry, multidisciplinary artist at the Invisible Dog Art Center, Brooklyn, NY**

We all have the power to choose our actions and responses. Harboring and expressing negative thoughts and feelings is one possible route. Another is to seek—and find—the positive, the silver lining, the path to healing and peace. *On the Way to Casa Lotus* shows the power of love and forgiveness, of listening closely to the knowing voice of our soul undeterred by outside opinions. It is an important reminder to all of the forgotten essentials in the quest for a peaceful, harmonious life.

—**Catharina Hedberg, owner, The Ashram**

On the Way to Casa Lotus is the deeply honest and vulnerable portrait of a young woman trying to juggle marriage and family in the midst of the severe depression, physical exhaustion, and debilitating pain resulting from a minor surgical procedure that turned into a long-term medical nightmare. But rather than focus on doctors' negligence or an impersonal medical system gone horribly off track, Junco Margain focuses on the personal growth, empowerment, and transformation this experience triggered. Her inconceivable journey, which begins in a place of low faith in her instincts, ultimately arrives at the most empowering stance only few who have been brutally victimized can take: genuine amnesty, self-acceptance, and forgiveness.

—**Renu Namjoshi, Ayurvedic counselor and Vedic astrologer**

ON THE WAY TO CASA LOTUS

ON THE WAY TO CASA LOTUS

A MEMOIR OF FAMILY, ART, INJURY, AND FORGIVENESS

Lorena Junco Margáin

On the Way to Casa Lotus: A Memoir of Family, Art, Injury, and Forgiveness
© 2021 Lorena Junco Margain

For information about special discounts for bulk purchases, please contact info@LorenaJuncoMargain.com.

Cuco Press
Austin, Texas
LorenaJuncoMargain.com

Printed in Canada.

Library of Congress Control Number: 2021900479
Hardcover ISBN: 978-1-7363905-0-4
Paperback ISBN: 978-1-7363905-1-1
Ebook ISBN: 978-1-7363905-2-8

Cover art: Jennifer Allora & Guillermo Calzadilla (JA 1975, GC 1971)
Shape Shifter, 2013
Sandpaper sheets glued on canvas
243.8 x 182.9 cm (96 x 72 inches)
Copyright Jennifer Allora & Guillermo Calzadilla
Courtesy of the artist and kurimanzutto, Mexico City / New York
Photo: Estudio Michel Zabé

Cover design by Kimberly Glyder / Interior design by Liz Schreiter
Editing and production by Reading List Editorial (readinglisteditorial.com)

Publisher's Cataloging-In-Publication Data
(Prepared by The Donohue Group, Inc.)

Names: Junco Margain, Lorena, author.

Title: On the way to Casa Lotus : a memoir of family, art, injury, and forgiveness / Lorena Junco Margain.

Description: [Austin, Texas] : Cuco Press, LLC, [2021]

Identifiers: ISBN 9781736390504 (hardcover) | ISBN 9781736390511 (paperback) | ISBN 9781736390528 (ebook)

Subjects: LCSH: Junco Margain, Lorena. | Mexican American women--Biography. | Women art collectors--Biography. | Surgical errors--Popular works. | Adrenal glands--Surgery--Popular works. | Forgiveness. | LCGFT: Autobiographies.

Classification: LCC E184.M5 J86 2021 (print) | LCC E184.M5 (ebook) | DDC 305.48/86872073092 B--dc23

*To the two constant forces
that have shaped my life:
family and art*

DEAR READER,

Welcome to Casa Lotus, home of my heart and heart of my home. For you to understand what I mean by this, it's important for you to know how I found my way here. My home at Casa Lotus is more than the sum of its parts: four walls and an oculus, brick and steel, art and water, love and toil. Casa Lotus is a lifestyle forged with intention, mindful joy, compassion for self, and respect for Mother Earth. Casa Lotus is the harmony that happens when outward decisions reverberate with inward consequence. What you put in your kitchen cabinet is what goes into your mouth. Electrical wiring zings with energy that is unseen but undeniably intimate, entering our eyes as light and our ears as music.

Everything that happened to me on my way to Casa Lotus laid the foundation for the life I live now and the life I hope to build in the future, just as the rugged road you are traveling on this moment is laying the foundation for all the possibilities of you. Every one of us has our own Casa Lotus, and we are all continually on our way. We must be gentle with our traveling selves. We must forgive the wind and rain that assail us as we go, always remembering that the harshest forces of nature (including human nature) carve beauty into everything, including ourselves.

I hope my story will reveal some part of the map that shows you the road to your own Casa Lotus. That place is there for you, I promise, and whether you realize it or not, you are already on your way.

With love and gratitude,

Lorena

PROLOGUE

On the way to Casa Lotus, the home I have imagined with my husband, Eduardo, the street bucks uphill and down, snakes left and right, and eventually sweeps a wide bend, shaped by one of the many small tributaries flowing into and out of the Colorado River. The Texas Hill Country is a watercolor landscape in early spring: muted amber, green, and gray. There's a halo of bluebonnets and wild flowers around the first blossoming redbud trees. Bright pops of red announce geraniums in terra-cotta pots outside the gates and garage doors. Palmettos and century plants occupy the flowerbeds, along with thick paddles of prickly pear cacti, determined to blossom and bear fruit, even in the crucible heat of a Texas summer.

Right now, Casa Lotus is a construction site, piled with bricks and lumber, mired in mud. But as I slog across the yard to the inlet where my children will swim someday, I think of Thich Nhat Hanh's book *No Mud, No Lotus: The Art of Transforming Suffering*. "If you don't have mud," he gently reminds us, "the lotus won't manifest. You can't grow lotus flowers on marble."

The opportunity to evolve past suffering and manifest joy has made me a work in progress. I get that, but there are days when I really wish we could jump the turnstile and go straight to the beauty. Casa Lotus and I are works in progress, but the house has begun to take shape. The structure is skeletal, but the metaphors are fully formed. Eduardo and I thought about this house carefully for eighteen months before we broke ground. With the help of many gifted architects, structural engineers, and artisans, we rendered precise drawings of every square foot and considered every detail, down to the native butterflies in the garden and the art in every room. I've curated every corner. The Spanish word *curación* means the same thing as the English word *curate*: to give cohesiveness to a body of work. But *curación* has an added layer of meaning: to disappear an illness, wound, or physical injury to a person. I grew up in Mexico with that tandem meaning in mind, and I love the idea that art does not simply fill a space; it brings wholeness to that space. Even when I was young, I had a feeling that love should work the same way, that we should curate the contents of our hearts and lives with the same mindful intention we would apply to a sculpture garden.

Studying art in college, I spent three consecutive summers in New York, and one day I happened to bump into Eduardo and his cousins on the street. I didn't know Eduardo well, but our parents and grandparents were friends in Monterrey. We came from the same social circle, but that wasn't the circle I wanted to be part of right then. I wanted to be a New Yorker, artsy and cool. Eduardo was dressed in preppy clothes, impeccably groomed and flawlessly well mannered.

We greeted each other, and he asked where I was going. I was on my way home, but I didn't want to feel obligated to invite him there, so I said, "Saks Fifth Avenue."

"Ah," said Eduardo. "That's where we're going."

His cousins seemed surprised to hear this since we were all on limited budgets.

"What a coincidence," I said.

"May we walk with you?"

"Of course."

What else was I going to say? I had to be polite, so off we went. Making small talk, we strolled up the street and went into the store.

"I assume you're going to the men's department. I'll go to ladies' and meet you back here in thirty minutes," I said. As soon as they walked away, I made my way through the store and slipped out the back door. And there was Eduardo, who had evidently had the same idea as me. We laughed, caught in the act.

"Where are you going now?" he asked.

"I'm…going to…church?"

"Why don't we go get a drink instead?"

I'd never noticed before that his eyes were so full of mischief.

This was not the day I met Eduardo, but it was the day we connected. We suddenly recognized each other, like when you arrive at a train station and see someone standing there with your name on a placard. *Oh, hello! You're my person. Let's get going, then.* I saw him fitting into my life the same way I see art fitting a certain space, and I trusted my instinct.

Early in our relationship, we visited my family's ranch near Monterrey, and while we were out canoeing, the boat capsized. Eduardo borrowed dry clothes from my brother, but I noticed at dinner that he was wearing his wet shoes. The shoes didn't fit him, and he was too proper to go without. *We'll have to work on that*, I said to myself. Eduardo brings me structure, and I'm the one who finally convinced him to go barefoot.

Family is everything in Mexican culture, and Eduardo is the contemporary version of the classic Mexican patriarch. He respects me as an equal but still insists on opening my car door. He's fiercely protective, but for the first ten years of our marriage, he operated on the comfortable assumption that I was strong enough to never need rescuing, and for the most part, this was true. He did his work, and I did mine. We traveled the world, and wherever we went I searched out the work of other artists I wanted to lift up. Together, we created our collection—a strong, worldly collection of more than a hundred works spanning a wide range of mediums, cultures, and contemporary voices from all over the globe.

With my partner Silvia, a dear friend since childhood, we founded an art gallery and cultural space in Monterrey, gathered Mexican art we planned to exhibit around the world, and gave talks on the concept of fair trade in the art world. I was eager to please, determined to be a good wife and mother and a force for good in the world, like my parents are.

My father (I call him Papi) is a remarkable man, the head of a remarkable family. Our family traditions are built around my parents' core ideal of unshakable integrity above all else. Papi is a firebrand who speaks his mind on whatever topic comes up at the dinner table. But he's also not afraid to exchange viewpoints with others, even to the extent that he devised a systemic approach to establishing editorial policies in the media institutions that he heads. In this system, the western concept of the ombudsman is taken one crucial step forward: not just to have a representative of the people in newsrooms but to have the people themselves! And not just anyone, but educated specialists, there pro bono, whose role is to question what information gets disseminated, ask hard questions, and make editorial decisions in different areas. Education, rule of law, energy, culture, sports, etc.—transparency and openness to the next level. It's a methodology that empowers community members to be professional—nonbiased—administrators of the information process. A voice that seeks the greater good: truth, ethics, responsible best practices. A nonviolent army of fifteen thousand community members that have gone out of their way over the course of three decades with the purpose of serving the information that impacts their communities and country. At the meeting of the American Newspaper Publishers Association, after hearing his talk on this model, more than one international media tycoon has approached him in disbelief: "I don't understand how you let these people meddle in your internal affairs." In a society that is typically hierarchical, it brings me pride and swells my heart every time erudite friends, experts in their field, approach me and share how participating in these editorial boards has enriched their lives. It's not just an idealistic model, but a way to expand the audience that values discernment in a world where information and ideology tear us apart. All of this makes some people like him and other people dislike him. My father receives both with the same stoic grace. Mami is the perfect partner for him. She supports his decisions without fail and plows the road for Papi in all things, big and small, planning great endeavors, playing with the grandchildren, and making his life function in so many ways.

I was born in Monterrey, and we moved to Mexico City when I was twelve. I grew up, studied art, married Eduardo. Our daughter Lore was born in 2006, and two years later, we were expecting another baby girl named Paty after Eduardo's mom.

Eduardo and I both love Mexico. The people are generous and full of joy. The art is vibrant and unafraid. The family-centered culture is in keeping with our own beliefs and priorities. But as the cities grew larger and larger all around us, Eduardo and I began to wonder if this was truly the best place to raise our children. When my parents announced that they were planning to move to the United States, we were torn. Eduardo was the breadwinner in our family, and his business was entirely centered in Mexico.

My family tends to flock, so ultimately Eduardo and I were swept along. We searched until we found houses on a pleasant cul-de-sac in Austin, where we could all live near one another. The children were thrilled because they would now be free to dash back and forth between houses while the mamas rocked babies on the porch swings and patios.

The circumstances of this move were beyond stressful. The decision to leave was abrupt, and within days, we were gone, but before we left, I insisted on one last visit to my OB, a good doctor with whom Eduardo and I had built a rapport. I was nervous about leaving him, leaving Mexico, leaving my friends and everything familiar.

"Do you believe in angels?" the OB asked.

This struck me as a very strange question to be asking, and I guess he could see that reaction on my face.

"You're leaving Mexico," he said, "but it will stay in your heart always. You have a difficult choice to make: stay in Monterrey with the increasing threats and risk your family's safety or go to the United States and do the work of making a new life there. Either way, you can close your eyes and summon an army of angels. Ask them to watch over your family, watch over the world. If you ask, they'll listen. They will deliver."

I do believe in angels, but I don't think of angels that way—like a great battalion of winged warriors in some Pre-Raphaelite painting or like the invariably fair-skinned seraphs who stare vacantly from the thatched roof of a nativity scene. When I need to summon my angels, I envision a bright white light, an aura that surrounds me and my family.

Austin was a strange and wonderful new world for me. I'd grown up sheltered under the wing of my close-knit family. I knew how to drive, but in mountainous Monterrey, I usually rode with sisters or friends. In Austin, I was happily tooling around at the wheel of a gloriously unremarkable white minivan, just like all the other moms. I pumped my own gas—a completely new experience—and shopped at the grocery and hardware stores.

In my garage studio, I continued creating the sort of multimedia installations that fascinated me, but now my work took on the added dimension of nesting. Our new home was a blank canvas. The creation of it was an ongoing process that brought together paint, fabric, stone, wood, and typography. In the foyer, I installed a parade of giant hammered brass ants that marched up the staircase wall. Enormous masterworks by my favorite artists brought a breath of Mexico into the living and dining rooms. I spent hours creating a display with several dozen colorful little round boxes from India. I attached the boxes to the wall (using the new drill I was thrilled to buy for myself at the hardware store) in a cloud that came up from the floor and swarmed around the corner. On white scrap paper, I wrote a good intention for each box.

Stay patient.

Speak your truth.

Be open.

I folded the paper, put it inside a box, and glued the lid on. It's still there today, my cloud of good intentions, and over the years, those scraps have whispered to me, reminding me that intention is there, whether we see it or not.

In accordance with tradition, I invited a priest to come and bless our new house. The smell of rosemary and hot wax drifted up to the high ceilings along with the familiar invocation, but as I followed him through the new house, the ritual echoed, as vacant and cold as the unfurnished rooms. He didn't know us like our priest in Monterrey did, so his prayers were the sort of generic one-Christ-fits-all invocations he would offer to anyone.

A few years later, I met a Colombian gentleman who was introduced to me as a spiritual healer. I mentioned the priest's visit and told him how the blessing had fallen flat for me.

"I felt guilty," I admitted. "I shouldn't have been so ungrateful. I wanted so much for our home to be happy and our baby healthy. The traditional words just didn't capture it."

"Your true intentions are worth more than any formal blessing," said the healer. "Perhaps you could think about what those silent prayers meant to you and act on that meaning."

I was still skeptical about this guy in general, but that idea did resonate. When I got home, I sat down with my daughters. Lore and Paty were five and three years old then. We folded little cards of glossy white paper and decorated the edges with glitter and glue, and assigned one card to each room in the house. Inside each card, we wrote a few words that captured the spirit of my intentions, a vision of the space and what our well-blessed life would look like there. I lit a candle and went from room to room with my precious little girls, reading the words out loud together.

Library: Knowledge, Encouragement, Foundations, Intrigue, Respect, Amazement—thinking of everything I wanted my children to take from a room full of books, maps, and art.

Bedroom: Rest, Peace, Healing, Intimacy, Growth—thinking of everything that happens when we sleep soundly and wake up revitalized.

Three years later, on a day when my life lay in ruins around me, I went to make myself a cup of tea, and when I opened the cupboard door, a little white card drifted down onto the countertop. I picked it up and stared at my own handwriting.

Kitchen: Nourishment, Sharing, Family, Friends, Love

The day we placed those cards, my heart was full of such good intentions. I had a busy calendar of things to do and places to be. I had good friends and a sense of purpose. The baseline joy in my life made it possible to navigate unpleasant surprises and stumbles without commotion or meltdowns. My body was strong and beautiful, and I devoted effort to keeping it that way. At a moment when my life was going well, I had tucked away that little blessing, thinking it was meant for my children. But Fate is playful. Turns out, it was a blessing for my future self. The little white card fluttered down into my hand on a day when I desperately needed to be reminded that life is rich with hidden gifts and secret messages. It was an urgent whisper.

Wake up! Listen to your body. You know who you are.

The story I'm about to tell you is true. If I had a knack for melodrama, I would keep you in suspense and peel the juicy tale like a blood orange, but when your life has actual drama in it, you lose your taste for melodrama, so I'll cut to the chase. When I was in my early thirties, I went to a well-respected surgeon to resolve a medical issue that was serious but not catastrophic—until the surgeon made a catastrophic mistake, destroyed my health, and left me with a lifetime of medical issues that can never be fully resolved and will likely take years off my life.

I've changed the name of the surgeon in these pages. I'm not afraid to name him—he's not Voldemort—but publicly shaming him would feel like revenge, and as I continue to rebuild my frail body and broken heart, I'm not willing to devote one teaspoon of my limited energy to vengeance. That said, I refuse to be a silent victim. I will not have my lips sutured shut. I feel compelled to share what I learned from living this nightmare. My father taught me by example the imperative of personal integrity, the great value and terrible cost of speaking the truth.

"The truth shall set you free," the Bible says, but that only happens when truth is spoken from a place of love. This is not the story of a bad person who ruined the life of a good person. It's the story of two good people whose destiny, in one devastating moment, connected like a fork and a light socket. Every one of us has the potential to be extraordinary one moment and faulty the next, because every one of us is uniquely human: fork today, light socket tomorrow. If we refuse to forgive, we do so at our own peril.

This is a love story, so it begins inside and moves outward, the way both love and stories do, the way art does, and babies, too.

All these precious things are invisible at first, hidden within, but impossible to contain. They grow, take on lives of their own, and go out into an unpredictable world, where good intentions occasionally meet with disaster. We are all human. Sooner or later, each of us will cross the path of someone who breaks our little world. You find yourself blindsided at an intersection, probably stuck for a while, unable to step over the wreckage. When you finally do summon the will to go on, you find two possible avenues before you. The road paved with resentment leads to bitterness. The road paved with forgiveness leads to healing.

I chose to forgive. I chose to learn. I chose to love. This book is about that choice, why I made it, and how it was tested.

Alexander Pope said, "To err is human, to forgive, divine." But forgiveness isn't some mystic power. It's a muscle you build by working it, and I started early. If I hadn't learned to forgive as a child, I would have had no friends. I was artsy and empathetic and wore my heart on my sleeve, which invited teasing in the best of circumstances and bullying in the worst. Long before I understood why, I could feel that my family was set apart from other people. As I grew up, I learned the dance of social expectations and witnessed the importance of gratitude, generosity, and humility.

In telling you my story, I hope to promote an ideology of forgiveness that makes room for both rage and redemption. I hope to show you a glimpse of forgiveness as a force for personal change—and for changing the world. My hope is to awaken those who ignore harsh truths about health care and surgical culture. I hope to validate and empower all those who suffer from an invisible or unnamed illness.

I hope, I hope. Because I am still human, still an optimist, even though this experience left me forever changed. What was done to me cannot be undone by myself or any surgeon. All I can do now is make peace with it and move on, planting a fresh blessing between the pages of this book, hoping that you, my friend, will find it.

one

In 2001, while Eduardo and I were planning our wedding, we went to see the movie *Moulin Rouge*. Remember the lush version of Elton John's "Your Song" in that movie? The strings take wing, Ewan McGregor sweeps Nicole Kidman out the window to dance across clouds, and the Man in the Moon, voiced by Plácido Domingo, sings them into Heaven. Tears stung my eyes. I gripped Eduardo's hand in the dark.

"This is our song," I said. "We must dance to it at the wedding."

And we did. It was perfect, arranged for strings and opera singers just like the movie version, and as I danced this first dance with my new husband, I felt the power of those words.

And you can tell everybody . . .

Isn't that precisely what a wedding is? Professing loudly, proudly, and in public: "My love and I are *we* now. Whatever comes next—joys and burdens, sickness and health—it's ours to share." I wanted our wedding to be a powerful statement about what Eduardo and I would be as a family.

My dress was made by Reem Acra. Flipping through the pages of *Vogue*, I'd seen a spectacular gown that featured a rebozo (pronounced *ray-BO-zo*), a long swath of colorful fabric Mexican women wear a thousand different ways. The rebozo might be wrapped around a woman's head to keep her wild hair in order and protect her neck from the sun while she's riding a horse or working in her garden. It can be wrapped around her torso to hold a baby to her breast or draped in whatever ingenious way accentuates her body and makes her feel beautiful. To me, it made the white wedding dress more worldly, more Mexican, and more me.

The funny footnote to this is that I visited Reem Acra in New York sixteen years later, and when I mentioned the wedding dress she'd made for me, she said, "Oh, yes! I remember. The first time I was in *Vogue*, they came and told me, 'This girl wants the dress from the picture,' but it didn't exist! I had just thrown a piece of fabric around the model's waist."

We laughed, but I thought about it for a long time. To Reem, the reality was pins and needles and a hurried moment in the studio, but when I saw that photograph, I saw a thousand years of history and purpose. The artist doesn't always know what she's creating, because art as an experience—like love as an experience—is created in equal parts by the one who gives and the one who receives. It's the chemistry of spontaneity and the courage to act on instinct, so the rebozo was perfect for me in ways I didn't even understand until years later.

For our tenth anniversary in 2011, Eduardo and I went on a motorcycle trip to Vegas. Romantic soul that he is, he took me to an Elton John concert. We were the lucky couple chosen to go up on stage when he sang "Your Song." We sat on the piano bench with him and took a prehistoric selfie with my old clamshell phone, but this was before the cloud, so when the phone died, the photo died with it. That moment in Vegas felt like a full circle, but years later I would realize that it was just the first arc of a journey much broader than either of us could imagine back then.

We both meant it when we swore to love each other "in sickness and in health." What a luxury it is to not know the true meaning of those words! But what a luxury to know what we know now, having been through all that we've been through together. It's the polarity of life, the extreme north and south, that builds history into a marriage as it evolves.

Still in my midtwenties, I felt invincible, the way young people do—until the birth of my first baby. I was naïve when I was pregnant with our little Lorenita. She didn't want to come out, and my contractions weren't enough to push this little bird from the nest. Finally, the doctor said the amniotic fluid was low. He had to do an emergency C-section, which is a bad moment to find out you're allergic to latex. The catheter caused my body to swell up like a beached whale. I lay there in misery upon misery, wanting to hold my baby and care for her, frustrated that I couldn't be her everything the way my mother was always everything for me. It was humbling to accept that I needed extra arms to help me be the mother I wanted to be.

"Mami," I finally admitted, choking back tears, "I need a nurse for the baby."

She and my mother-in-law, Patricia (but I call her Tía Paty), set to work interviewing candidates who might fit into the unusual world of my family. Someone who would actually be part of my family.

"I found the perfect nurse," Mami told me, and a few days later, I met Blanca—my right arm and guardian angel to this day. She had a broad smile that lit up her eyes, but her teeth were an example of the way things are done too often in Mexico. Whatever the problem is, pulling the tooth seems to be the go-to solution. Blanca was (and still is) a treasure. Her invaluable services were a gift from Mami for the first three months, and as we drew closer to the time when she would leave, Eduardo said, "I don't care if it takes half my salary. We can't lose her."

I needed her to stay healthy, so I helped her have her unstoppable smile reconstructed and, in a poetic twist, helped her daughter go to college to become an orthodontist. Blanca is family to us. There's no challenge too big for her. Whatever it is, she'll figure it out. She has courage that I've never seen in anyone else, and when my own courage runs dry, she lends me some.

Two years later, together Blanca and I cared for my second baby, named Paty, honoring her grandmother, who had four boys. She helped me create a home for my family while I continued my work as an artist and as a curator for my galleries and traveling exhibits. We invented a unique partnership. She made it possible for me to do everything I needed to do, and I made it possible for her to reinvent her life, send her children to college, and make sure they owned homes of their own. She moved to Texas with us when I was pregnant with Paty and through the difficult years that followed, always keeping the bedtime and bath time traffic moving, putting healthy food on the table, and lavishing special attention on whatever child needed it at any given moment. When I was feeling strong, she was my right hand, and when my strength left me, she was everything. Neither of us could have anticipated what lay ahead.

In spring 2012, when I was pregnant with our third child, Eddie Jr., my little sister Roby was diagnosed with thyroid cancer. She was four months pregnant, happily awaiting a new baby. The diagnosis itself was alarmingly swift. One morning she woke up with a cough. The doctor told her she had a sinus infection, but when he examined her neck, his fingers grazed a lump just above her collarbone. He immediately sent her for a biopsy, which revealed cancer of the thyroid.

The news hit our family like a thunderbolt. Poor Mami wailed as if her heart had been laid open. Roby was instantly in crisis mode, and everyone in the family mobilized to support her. My little sister needed me, and I would be there for her. There was no room for my fear, no time for me to be weak. I could not be sick right now. In an instant, everything troubling me was set aside. All my thoughts, all my heart, everything was about Roby now. It was not my turn to need help. Roby needed all of us to be strong for her, and poor Mami was so distraught, I worried almost as much for her as I did for my sister. My father made sure that Roby had the best possible care, and our mother thought of everything—for Roby and for the baby—keeping her as calm and comfortable as possible.

My sister's team quickly came together—oncologist, radiologist, obstetrician—and surgery was scheduled to remove her thyroid. It was terrible to sit there waiting for several weeks, knowing that the cancer was advancing, but her doctors wanted to give her the best chance of getting through the surgery without losing the baby. Roby was four months pregnant when she was diagnosed. She needed to be five months along, giving the baby's organs the opportunity to develop, so that if she went into labor during surgery, the baby girl might still survive. She and I stuck close by each other as the weeks went by, watching our bellies get bigger and bigger.

The surgery went smoothly, and the baby stayed right where she belonged. Surrounded by love, Roby recovered from the surgery and pressed on through the remaining months of the closely monitored pregnancy without her thyroid. When the day came for her to deliver, I posted up in a recliner next to her hospital bed. I was coping with the sort of hernia common to pregnant women (the bulk of the baby pushes a section of intestine through the weakened wall of stretched muscle), so my OB had ordered bed rest for the final five months. We lay there, side by side, keeping each other's spirits up, though we groaned and pressed our palms to our bellies when we laughed. Whenever a new nurse came on duty, she had to ask, "Wait—which one of you is having the baby today?"

Mami was not able to be there, because her mother—our mystical, delightful, vivacious grandmother—was dying in Mexico. Our *abuela* was so full of life, it was impossible for me to accept the fact of her death. She was widowed young, so she'd known loss of her own, but she was an innately joyful being—offbeat and adventurous, with her own free-spirited way of doing things. Accordion band for Christmas? Why not! She was a sensual being, beautiful, and worldly wise, with flame-red hair and big eyes.

In contrast, my mother is an understated beauty. She's every bit as elegant and bold as my grandmother, every bit as creative, but she wears it the way a magnolia tree wears its graceful limbs. From her I've learned a thousand little things about how to create a lovely home and be a gracious host. My mom is a visionary, and she helped me see things in a creative light.

My mother is my rock-solid counterpoint, the one I turn to for strength and balance anytime I need a reality check. My grandmother was my playful familiar, the one I could count on to validate my unconventional side. The loss of her left me reeling. It made me think about the loss of my mother, and that's a thing I can't bear to contemplate.

Roby and I could spare no energy for grief at that moment. We had to look to the future and let go of the past. The day our grandmother died, Roby gave birth to a beautiful baby girl, and soon after that, in August 2012, Eduardo and I welcomed our baby boy into the world. As soon as he was out and accounted for, I was taken to the OR for surgery to repair the hernia.

The doctor who performed the surgery was lanky and confident, not just tall, but basketball-player tall with great, graceful hands and a kindly bedside manner. I'm going to call him Dr.

Humano, because whatever else he is or is not, he turned out to be all too human.

The surgery went smoothly, and I went home to my family. Holding our healthy babies in our arms, my sister and I laughed and cried. Like the psalmist said, "Weeping endures through the night, but joy comes in the morning." What a thing to go through! My God. It was terrible, but here at the end was sweetness.

I was eager to regain my strength and take on the world again. I expected my body to rebound the way it did after Lore and Paty were born. I waited eagerly for that burst of nesting energy, but it never came. I waited for the spinning wheel of my mind to produce a clean straight thread, but the tangled knots of grief and fear were still there as I woke up every morning and lay down every night.

People kept telling me, "Be patient. Give it some time." I consulted Dr. Google, searching keywords like *postpartum fatigue* and *baby blues*. A month went by, then two months, then three. A frightening realization began to form like a spider web in the corner of my mind.

There's something wrong with me.

two

After little Eddie was born, Eduardo and I bought a condo on the beach in South Padre Island, a pleasant town on a barrier island in the Gulf of Mexico just north of the border. It's a short flight from Austin and even shorter from Monterrey, so many of our friends and family vacationed there as well. We envisioned a place where we could retreat from the world and be together as a family, a place where it was safe for the children to ride their bikes along the boardwalk, play for hours on the beach, go for burgers, and forge strong bonds with their cousins. It takes a village to raise a child, right? So we made our own little village right there on the beach, and it became our family sanctuary.

Sitting on the sand with my sisters, watching our children play in the water, I cherished each moment of gossip and laughter. It reminded me of the way we were when we were kids. We hadn't changed much, really. My oldest sister was still direct and intelligent. I, the middle sister, was still idealistic and always trying too hard. Roby was still our baby, bold and humorous. Our big brother's wife, my sister-in-law, was fully one of our own, inventive and kind, always looking out for everyone. They knew something was off, that I wasn't quite myself since Eddie was born, but we were all still reeling a bit from the loss of our *abuela* and the shock of Roby's cancer.

"Give it time," Mami kept saying. "Give it time."

So I gave it time. I sat in the sun with my sisters and said nothing. I didn't know what to say. I wasn't actively ill in a way that I could present to a doctor, checking off boxes and filling in blanks, but I knew some aspect of my body was not fully operational. Like fog rolling in off the water, the symptoms crept into my life quietly, barely above a whisper at first, so it was easy for me to ignore my gut instincts, blame myself, chalk it up to extra weight or weakness, focus on caring for others instead of feeling sorry for myself. When I tried to express my growing concern to Eduardo or Mami or my sisters, I always censored myself. I didn't want to sound like I was whining.

Since I was a child, everyone has told me, "Oh, Lorena, you're too sensitive." When I was little, they said it was because I was a girl, and later on, they blamed my "artistic nature." There's a natural tendency, I think, to distance ourselves from that which makes us uncomfortable. Helplessness is uncomfortable, so when someone who loves you is confronted with the fact of your pain and their own inability to fix it, their knee-jerk reaction is to push it away. *No*, they tell themselves, *it can't be that bad*. That would be too awful. They don't want that for you. They need to believe you're okay. They need the problem to be your sensitivity, not something frightening, unknown, and unfixable.

This comes from a place of love, which doesn't change the fact that it's irritating. It's better than thinking they genuinely don't care, which is almost never the case, but either way, it's isolating. There's nothing lonelier than an undiagnosed illness, a hidden malady that has no name but casts an undeniable shadow. There's no liberating "you can tell everybody" feeling. You can't tell anybody, because you have no claim to the vocabulary of diagnosis. Words like *cancer*, *diabetes*, and *brain tumor* instantly create a context for compassion and understanding. Without any such words, I felt I was left alone in an uncomfortable silence as my vibrant world gradually turned gray, but all my issues shrank to insignificance when I compared them to what my little sister was going through. When I struggled to get out of bed in the morning, I badgered myself, *Shut up, Lorena. It's not like you have cancer.*

Something I wish I had understood at the time—one of the many lessons I took away from this whole disastrous year—is that comparing your suffering to someone else's suffering is worse than apples to oranges. It's apples to elephants. Your suffering has its own paradigm. It's not made smaller by someone else's suffering or made greater by someone else's healing. You don't get extra credit if your disease has a worse diagnosis than someone else's, and you aren't obligated to keep your little chin up just because your brand of suffering lacks a trending hashtag or colorful ribbon.

Your suffering is whatever it is *to you*. No more, no less. Perhaps your ribbon is invisible. You're still bound by it.

Several months after Eddie was born, I still wasn't feeling like my prepregnancy self. I was too busy to think about it most of the time, but my energy was off. Fatigue frayed the edges of everything I wanted to do until I really didn't want to do anything anymore. My thoughts and emotions felt blunted. I couldn't articulate this sensation that accumulated on my brain and body like a layer of late-summer dust.

One day when my daughters were at school, my mother took Eddie Jr. so I could have a little time to myself. It troubled her that I was feeling so low, but because she loves me, she wanted to believe that it was the usual postpartum fatigue. I wanted to believe she was right. I clung to the idea until I couldn't anymore. That day, I walked through my quiet studio, surveying the possibilities of paint, pastels, and blank canvases. Industrial materials begged to be bent and shaped. Chunks of quartz and cracked geodes waited for me to make sense of their hidden potential. I felt the call of every work in progress, but that part of my spirit that used to call back to them was gone.

Stepping over a little installation Paty had made over the weekend, a circle of rocks and flowers that echoed work she'd seen me do, I examined a piece I'd been working on for months. Pouring wax over a large seashell, I had observed how it morphed into an entirely different being as all its jagged edges turned soft and muted. I had let the wax cool and cure, poured again, let it cool and cure, poured again. Looking back now, I see that it was me I was making: an organic being encased in layer upon layer of smooth, suffocating fatigue, fogginess of thought, deep muscle weakness, and an even deeper depression. Each new symptom poured over me, cooling, curing, changing the composition of my nature.

Before Eddie Jr. was born, Silvia and I were mounting the *Shaped in Mexico* exhibit at a gallery in London. We collected this array of disparate works and engaged with the artists with all the intensity I felt when I was studying and creating art in college. Now I looked at them and felt only a tepid, utilitarian sort of interest. Among them was a strangely provocative painting of a bone, pale colors on a white background, that beautifully captured an inner universe of patterns and landscapes. When I bought this painting, I was impressed with the execution and composition. Now it spoke to me about the intimate wisdom of my own body. I was ready to say it: *There's something wrong with me.*

I called the office of the OB/GYN who had delivered Paty and Eddie Jr. and told the receptionist, "I would like an appointment to speak with Dr. García."

"This is a well-woman exam?"

"No exam," I said. "I want to talk to him in his office."

It took some effort to make her understand that no, I was not in pain, and yes, the baby was fine. I had no symptoms to report. I wanted to have a conversation that didn't begin with "lie back and open your legs." I didn't want to be spread-eagle on a paper-covered table while he took notes with his back to me. This was a conversation about my *self*, not just my body. I chose to see Dr. García because he'd known me for years. He was familiar with my history and the intimate landscape of my body, and just as important, he understood the dynamics of my family and the culture I came from. I needed him to understand and believe me when I told him, upright and eye to eye, "Something is wrong."

I felt the difference the moment I sat down across from him.

"Hello, Lorena," he said. "What a nice surprise."

"Hello, Mario," I said.

I feel perfectly comfortable using a doctor's first name. Why shouldn't we? I find it odd that patients so often say "Dr. So-and-so" while a doctor calls them by their first name. It's not like we were teacher and student. We were equals, seated in proper chairs with a desk between us, collaborating in a scientific investigation. That's the reality of any appointment you have with your doctor. He is a consultant you have hired because he has the expertise to interpret data and make observations. Ideally, it's a friendly collaboration, and at the very least, I have learned, it has to be mutually respectful.

"And how is Eduardo?"

"He's good. Still commuting. He comes home on Friday afternoon and leaves early Monday morning. We miss him, but he needs to be in Monterrey for work."

"Do you think about moving back?" he asked.

"No, Austin is home now. We want the children to grow up here."

"How is the baby?"

"Almost eight months old," I said. "Can you believe it?"

He smiled, looking at me expectantly, patiently waiting for me to get to the point.

"Something I've noticed," I said, "is the differences between the medical systems in the US and Mexico."

"Such as . . ."

"Well, one example that says so much—the hospital rooms don't have extra chairs for family. They don't expect you to arrive with an entourage. In Mexico, the hospital room has an extra bed. They know your family wouldn't leave you to spend the night alone."

He laughed and nodded. "So true. So true. It's not right for Abuela to arrive for her visit and have no bed."

"That would be appalling!" I laughed, too, but then I said seriously, "In Mexico, doctors call you, no matter how late in the evening, to share test results. They know you're waiting and worrying. They return calls and texts. They follow up. They listen. Lately, I have not experienced that here."

"Also true." He folded his hands on his desk. "Lorena, I did do all that for a while after I came to the United States six years ago. It led to my divorce."

"How so?"

"My family was not always my first priority. It caused a rift."

"I'm sorry," I said. His candor was another unexpected equalizer.

"It may seem that doctors in the US are more distant," he said, "but the plain truth of the matter is, they have their own problems—their own lives."

"But aren't they here to heal?"

"Of course, but they have to help as many people as they can."

"I keep thinking that if I went to Mexico for treatment—"

"Treatment for what?"

"I don't know! That's why I'm here. People keep saying it's because I had another baby or because I'm worried about my parents or missing Eduardo. They blame it on circumstances, but I know—*I know*—something is not right. I can't explain it. I don't have any real symptoms."

"What do you mean by 'real' symptoms?"

"Something that's obviously wrong. A fever, a cough, a broken bone."

"Just tell me how you feel."

"I feel . . . weak, maybe? Anxious. Uncomfortable. Like everything is upside down. My heart is too fast, and my legs are too slow. I can't concentrate on a book. Creating art always made me excited and frustrated and joyful all at once. Now I don't feel anything."

He nodded, so very knowing, so very understanding. "Lorena, many women go through this. You've had a major surgery along with the new baby. Your *abuela* passed away. It's been a tough year. Naturally, you're feeling somewhat depressed."

"No. It's not depression. It's something physical."

He sighed again and pressed for specifics—chest pain, numbness, tingling, insomnia—but I couldn't offer anything concrete. Why was I even here? I couldn't answer my own questions, much less his.

"Lorena, I'm going to prescribe an antidepressant for you," he said. "Just to help you through the next few months. You'll see. This will pass, and you'll be your old self again. It's nothing to worry about."

"I would prefer not to take anything like that," I said, but it sounded meek, even to me. "I don't think it's going to help."

"You might be surprised." He jotted something on my chart and thumb-clicked a pen over his prescription pad. "Imagine you're at a funeral. Everyone is grieving, dressed in black. You take these, and you're still at the funeral, but all you see are the beautiful flowers. The problems don't disappear, but you feel hopeful again. You're able to enjoy this beautiful world you live in."

It sounded so easy. I was tempted to believe it. Maybe it was possible to pour a smooth coat of wax over whatever was troubling me, but the jagged edge would still be there inside me. I might *feel* fine, but I wouldn't actually *be* fine. I searched out a second opinion—and a third and a fourth—and every doctor told me the same thing: "Take a few of these pills and you'll feel fine." In medical school, doctors are taught "When you hear hoofbeats, think horses, not zebras." It's a sensible approach until they apply it to a patient with invisible stripes.

Does it count as depression, I wondered, *if I'm depressed about the way people keep insisting that I'm depressed?*

One day as I was waiting for Lore after gymnastics, I noticed another mom reading a book called *Change Your Brain, Change Your Life* by Daniel G. Amen. I asked her about it and was intrigued enough to stop at a bookstore on my way home. That night I sat up late, reading about how the brain triggers anxiety and depression and how it can be reprogrammed for dramatic change. When Eduardo came home, I told him all about it.

"The author is a neuropsychiatrist," I said. "I booked an appointment at his clinic in New York. The website says they can scan your brain and identify problem areas."

"Problem areas?" He sounded skeptical.

"I'm going," I said. "Maybe this is the answer I've been looking for."

"I'll go with you," said Eduardo.

"There's no need. I won't be gone long. Two days for the appointment, and maybe I'll stop by a few galleries."

"I'd like to come with you."

I wanted to do this on my own, but he was adamant. We flew to New York together a few days later. The first day at the clinic, I filled out an extensive questionnaire about my mental and physical health and my medical history. A nurse started an IV to flush my system with radioactive contrast solution for the brain scan. Sitting in front of a computer screen, I performed a series of tasks designed to stimulate specific parts of my brain.

"Match these shapes," said the doctor's assistant.

I tried hard to focus. I wanted to be perfect, 100 percent.

"Tap the cursor when you see the line move."

I felt a satisfying sense of accomplishment every time I tapped. I was getting it right.

"Now we'll go next door for the scan," the technician told me. "It's a little like taking an athlete's blood pressure after she runs a mile. The mental exercises stimulate activity in your brain. Tomorrow, we'll use meditation and music to calm brain activity and repeat the scans so we can do a comparison. We'll be able to see all sorts of interesting things."

"And you'll have the results right away?"

"Oh, yes. We'll go over everything before you leave."

I lay still for the scan, breathing, holding my breath, breathing again, feeling the same proactive sense of direction. Instead of taking the antidepressants, I was doing the work to figure out what was wrong, get the diagnosis for the underlying issue, and fix it.

In the waiting room afterward, I looked around for Eduardo, but he wasn't there. I thought he'd probably stepped out for coffee, so I called his cell, but there was no response. I asked after him at the front desk, and the receptionist said, "He's gone for his scan."

"Excuse me?"

"He wanted to have it done, and we were able to work him into the schedule," she said with a smile. "He's very persuasive."

"Yes," I said dryly. "I know."

"He should be done in thirty minutes or so."

I waited for an hour, feeling like a bride who's been upstaged by the maid of honor. This diagnosis meant a lot to me. I had hinged all my hope on it. I needed it to provide the life-changing answer

I'd been searching for. To my skeptical spouse, apparently, it was a game.

When he came out, he was all smiles, even when I glared and asked, "Why are you doing this?"

"We came all this way." He shrugged. "I figured I might as well. That was pretty cool, wasn't it?"

"Cool?"

"Hey, I'm starving. Let's go get dinner."

Deep breath, Lorena. Just breathe, I told myself. He was being protective in the only way he could. He suspected the whole thing was a scam, and the only way to know was to subject himself to the same procedure they were giving me. This was not how I wanted him to participate—in fact, I hadn't wanted him to participate at all—but I was willing to give him points for good intentions. This mysterious illness was uncharted territory for me, and supporting a wife with a mysterious illness was uncharted territory for him. We would have to cut each other some slack in order to get through this.

Over dinner, we compared notes. We'd each been asked to fill out the same questionnaire—a lengthy list of "on a scale of 0 to 5" evaluations—that would compare my assessment of my current symptoms with Eduardo's perception of my current symptoms. The disparity in our answers made me laugh.

Do you experience anxiety when attending a party?

I looked at that and thought of everything from food to foundation garments. Who wouldn't feel a minimum level 3 anxiety about all that? But I am good at social functions, so Eduardo, who was used to seeing me dressed to the nines, working the room, and dancing the night away, looked at the same question and confidently checked me in at 0 anxiety. It's a case of Instagram Syndrome. Not everyone who looks like they're having a wonderful time is actually having a wonderful time.

The next day, we returned to the clinic for our second set of scans. I let my mind drift and settle with the meditation music and lay still, contrast solution rushing through my veins. When I sat down with the doctor to go over the results, he showed me a splayed Rorschach-type image, a rich tapestry of indigo, gray, and red on black.

"Here you see the active view, and this all looks very healthy," he said. "A lot of activity in the cerebellum, just as it should be with the concentration exercises."

He put up an image that looked like a mushroom from a *My Little Pony* cartoon, a soft blob of pastel purple, pink, and chartreuse.

"It's . . . pretty," I said.

"The surface view here, looking down from the top, looks nice and symmetrical. We're looking at the shape here, not the colors." He went back to the active view. "Interesting. Your brain is actually more lit up when you're relaxed."

"Is that abnormal?"

"It's less common, but nothing to worry about."

I studied the muted rainbow in my brain, trying to think of the right questions to ask while he made notes on my chart.

"Overall, your brain looks wonderful," he concluded. "Beautiful, really."

"What does that mean, in terms of a diagnosis?"

"It means you're fine," he said. Like he was planting a flag on top of a mountain. *Congrats! You're fine!* And then he handed me the paperwork in a way that felt like a firm nudge toward the door.

So Eduardo was right to be skeptical. I assumed he would get a "diagnosis" identical to mine, and then we'd know it was all *mierda*—a load of BS—but when I met him in the hallway, he was peering at his paperwork, brows furrowed.

"What did they tell you?" I asked.

"It's not so good. My brain is too active. They gave me a wellness treatment and a prescription for GABA, a neurotransmitter. It's supposed to calm me down. What did they tell you?"

"He said I'm fine."

I turned away, and Eduardo followed me down the hall to the elevator.

"Lorena, you should be glad." He set his arm around my shoulders and pulled me close. "This is good news. Your brain is healthy. Why are you so upset?"

"I'm fine."

Fine. I was fine. Other than feeling like a madwoman, other than feeling like my body had been wrung out like a mop, other than my emotions slowly turning to quartz, yes, I was just fine.

We flew home, and that night, facing myself in the bathroom mirror, I twisted the childproof cap from the bottle of antidepressants and tapped a blue caplet into the palm of my hand. I didn't feel the proactive buzz of energy I'd felt when I was pursuing that elusive diagnosis. I felt overwhelmed by the heaviness of my heart.

Maybe they were all right, and I was wrong. Maybe I was fine and just needed to see the flowers. A towering fortress of disbelief surrounded me, and only one doorway had been offered, so every night for the next several weeks, I swallowed the recommended daily dosage, wanting to believe everyone else instead of myself.

You're fine. You're fine. You're fine.

Of course, I wasn't. But that didn't seem to matter.

three

After a few weeks on antidepressants, I was certain there was no such thing as a pill that makes you see only flowers, and if there is, I didn't want it.

Look around you at a funeral. You see love. You see family. You see life going on with all its joys and sorrows. Yes, of course, I was still reeling from the death of my *abuela* and the birth of my son, but how could it be unhealthy to feel the full depth of that sorrow and the full height of that challenge? If anything, I wanted to feel more, not less, and the persistently stony feeling in my soul was still there, along with a host of subtle physical symptoms that left me feeling achy and fatigued.

One morning, after taking the girls to school, I was sitting in the kitchen and experienced a surrealistic moment when I suddenly felt as if I were sinking into my chair. The cushion underneath me felt like quicksand. My body felt like it was made of cinder block. I tried to concentrate on a running list of things I should be doing—making Lore's costume for a school play, researching holiday travel plans, calling vendors about an upcoming event at an art gallery—but I couldn't focus my thoughts.

Looking around the kitchen, through a haze of dust motes in the sunlight, all I could see was a layer of grime. The staff had cleaned every surface that morning. I'd watched them mop the floors and wipe the countertops. Why was it so filthy? How would I capture all these particles in the air? What was that greasy film that coated the baseboards? Soap bubbles had left pockmarks on the sink. There were crumbs on the table—no, *clumps* on the table. Blobs of food and filth. The walls were warped and teeming with bacteria. I knew this was delusional. My home was pristine.

I forced myself out of my chair and stumbled to the pantry, searching the shelves for a bottle of hand sanitizer, but I couldn't find it. I ransacked the drawers in the kitchen and the medicine cabinet in the bathroom. *Finally!* Thank God. Here. I found a small plastic bottle of pale blue gel. The gel felt cold and clean between my hands. I felt calmer, but still confused. What was I looking for? What was I supposed to be doing?

I kept thinking of my grandmother. She was so much fun to be around, always full of sass and mischief. My siblings and I always stayed with her when our parents were traveling, which was often. She took us swimming and hiking and showed us the hidden worlds inside the rocks and geodes she collected. I was glad to be tall, like her, and my body type wasn't the only strength I'd inherited from her. I felt her proud spirit lift my head up whenever some kid at school made me feel low.

Nothing felt right after Abuela left us. Nothing was where it belonged. She should be here. I should have been at her funeral. During the last days of her life, Roby, my baby sister, and I were pregnant. More than anything, Abuela wanted to live to see the new babies. Now they would grow up never having seen her face.

I made myself a cup of tea and sat down at the table to drink it. Suddenly, I felt myself drift upward. I was not sleeping. My eyes were wide open. This was not a dream. I drifted above the ceiling and beyond. I was in my grandmother's bedroom. All the family was gathered around her. There was peace in this moment, in this space. It felt good to remain suspended there, but suddenly, I was back in my chair. In the kitchen. The busy clang of pots and pans set my teeth on edge. I couldn't stay with that peaceful moment, but the moment stayed with me, comforting and disturbing at the same time.

Weeks passed, and I felt weirdly unwell, but I forced myself to set one foot in front of the other, doing what had to be done each day. Doctors agreed there was nothing wrong with me, but I felt like a burden to everyone so I just silenced myself. There were other issues to be concerned about.

Priorities, Lorena.

When I was growing up in Mexico, I never experienced a moment of doubt: Papi and Mami valued family above all. Nothing was more important to them than their children. But even as children, we knew that our father cared for all people and felt compelled to help wherever he could. I understood, even as a child, that what's most important isn't always most immediate. This was the hierarchy of values I was raised with: integrity is paramount, but when your family needs you, you set everything else aside, even yourself.

I learned from my parents and grandmother that it was the responsibility of every single member of society to do good—to be good—and use whatever gifts God has given us to make the world a better place. If you are loved, it was your responsibility to love others without judgment. If you have received good things in your life, then it was your turn to pay it forward and share with others less fortunate. If you've been heard, it's your responsibility to speak up on behalf of those who can't speak up for themselves.

When I began to make my way in the world as an artist, I had such a fire in my belly. I wanted to make my creative voice heard, and I knew there were many other artists who felt that need as deeply as I did. I felt a kinship with my fellow creators and wanted to amplify their voices. At the same time, I felt a kinship with those who hunger for art and see it as an essential element of their life and home.

A vision of how to bring the two together had begun to take shape. Creating art in the form of a home, art in the shape of a life, art that lives and breathes with a family. This vision could become something of a business, I was certain. I hoped to build something that mattered every bit as much as the businesses built by the men in my family.

I was almost there, close enough to reach out and get my hands around it.

But in the weeks that followed Roby's surgery, it seemed as though a shadow had been cast across my body. The vision withered and went dormant before it had a chance to flower.

four

Roby looked stronger and more beautiful every time I saw her. After the baby was born, she left the hospital with her bundle of joy, set to work rebuilding her body, and moved on with her life. Problems solved, for the moment. I'm sure it didn't feel so simple as that when she was going through it, but on a fundamental level, that's how you get answers. You show up with a palpable lump. The biopsy is marked *stat*. The right questions are asked, and when the answer is cancer, everything jumps into hyperdrive. Professionals follow protocol. Family and friends snap to attention. A rush of adrenaline powers everyone through the crisis, and when the crisis has passed, everyone is eager to get back to normal.

The diagnostic journey doesn't always follow such a clear trajectory, and it's never Point A to Point B, when endocrinology is concerned. Our bodies are exquisitely complex, every system interplaying with another. Our adrenal glands, tiny but powerful, wield a profound influence on our physical and emotional well-being. They produce hormones that control heart rate, blood pressure, and metabolism of vital nutrients, plus chemical triggers that spark the stress response—the fight-or-flight instinct—and a host of other autonomic responses constantly coming and going below the surface of conscious thought, a vast, invisible ecosystem that makes life sustainable and experiences meaningful. Because the influence of the adrenal glands is felt throughout the body and mind, it's hard to connect the dots between symptoms and an adrenal gland gone wrong.

So, for me, there was no such thing as normal. Normal was a distant memory. An illusion. I felt hollow and tired, and I couldn't understand why. My doctor told me I was fine, so I blamed myself. I focused on my children, my family, charity work, the artists I sought out and supported, pushing through each day, weighted by thick fatigue and sadness. My head pounded the dull rhythm of my pulse. My body ached on what felt like a cellular level. I continued taking the antidepressants the OB/GYN had prescribed, but I actively sought answers beyond the little blue pills, which could have been lemon drops, for all the good they did.

In my quest for physical and emotional healing, I consulted doctors, naturopaths, and advisors (some more helpful than others) and read everything I could. I wanted a word—*any word*. I wasn't asking for something easy, just something quantifiable, something to fill in a blank, check a box on a chart. Schedule a surgery. Cut me up. Rearrange my insides. Make me whole again. With an answer in hand, I could face whatever came next. When it seemed like there was no answer, I began to despair, thinking there was no fix for this and that anyone who claimed to have that silver bullet cure-all was a liar.

There was bitterness that came with this realization, but my search for a solution had a strange side effect. I discovered that almost everyone around me was searching for an answer of their own. As I became more at ease with the conversation, talking with other moms at school or strangers in waiting rooms, I could see that every one of us is imperfect, feeling a bit broken, going a little crazy. Every one of us is searching, and every one of us has some little clue to follow, some small piece of the treasure map. The only way to see the big picture is to share our stories. It's scary to let others in on the terrible truth that our lives are not the perfect lives we post on social media, but that simple admission is also freeing. Now the conversation is about solutions, coping mechanisms, and new pathways to investigate.

I was fascinated by the variety of belief systems around me. Some people are skeptical of anything other than doctor's orders. Others pray, though their faith is shaken. Others swear by a plant-based diet or colloidal mineral toddy or crystals in your pocket. I tend to be utilitarian about my beliefs; I believe in what works.

As an art major in college, I created an extended meditation on form and function for my senior thesis. I painted a 262-foot-long white carpet with gold-and-peach flowers and a border of green leaves. While I worked on this project, it seemed to stretch on for miles. For two weeks, I gave myself over to the seemingly endless pattern, the carefully measured details, and the perfect symmetry. The piece was an experience for me, a journey of discovery, an exercise in precision and patience. It crafted me as I crafted it. Together, I and my work of art evolved.

My mother shuffled the furniture from one of the bedrooms to clear a space where I could work on the enormous piece, and when I finally finished my work, she helped me roll it into a hefty bale. The chapel where Eduardo and I were about to get married is located by a countryside hacienda in Mexico. I lugged the carpet there and created an elaborate installation. Set against the religious symbology and traditional architecture, the piece became something entirely different. I placed a camera at one end, focusing on the carpet itself, filming only the feet that stepped on it—or declined to step on it—throughout our wedding day. The work evolved again and became a social experiment of sorts.

I wanted to see how people reacted to this work of art in contrast to a regular machine-made runner—handmade versus industrial—and perhaps draw some useful conclusions that might apply on a grander scale. If a city is filled with art and beauty, for example, might people tread a bit more carefully there?

When I looked at the footage (pardon the pun) from the long day of ceremony and celebration, observing the way people interacted with this work of art in the midst of all the food and dancing and socializing, I found that most people paused. Many knelt to touch the hand-painted flowers and run their fingers along the textured edges of the leaves. Some walked on it with obvious relish, as if the carpet made them lighter on their feet. The children were especially swept up, skipping and playing up and down this magical painted garden. Very few people were indifferent to it, the way you would be to a machine-made runner from a factory. There was an undeniable energy here that only a few people could tromp over without noticing.

It was a thing of beauty, but it had meaning, too, and part of this experiment was contemplating what that meaning was for me. It was a carpet, after all. The moment I rolled it out, I made it available to everyone at the wedding, and I as an artist had to accept that I had no control over anyone's choice to enjoy or utilize or avoid it in whatever way felt natural to them. I overheard a few interesting conversations about art in general and this art in particular. There was some speculation about significance, intent, and proper protocol when it comes to art that refuses to stay on the wall where most well-behaved art is consigned to live. Perhaps at the end of the day, the purpose of the piece was to provoke thought and ignite that sort of discussion, creating a figurative and literal pathway to understanding.

I imagine this may be what it feels like for anyone who seeks to inspire or teach others. Some people get it, and some people don't, and that's okay. If they don't get it, it wasn't meant for them, and if you don't get what they're saying about it, that's not meant for you. I lean toward the literal; whether the discussion is about herbal tea or the New Testament, my feeling is, if it works for me, I believe in it. If it doesn't resonate, I don't judge its value for someone else. Not everything has to resonate for every person, and even something that doesn't resonate for me might spur me to think differently about things that do. I can be inspired by someone whose idea of inspiration is totally different from mine.

All of which is to say: I keep an open mind.

During that stressful time after Roby's cancer experience, while I was groping through the darkness of my own nondiagnosis, my childhood friend, Valeria, invited me to go to a seminar given by Renu Namjoshi, a Vedic astrologer. Since almost everyone is familiar with the story of Steve Jobs, Renu used his chart as an example, pinpointing the planetary patterns that may have influenced his life.

"Valeria, I don't really believe in all that," I said. "Do you?"

She shrugged her strong shoulders, open to whatever, and I figured, *Hey, who am I to second-guess the universe?* At this point, I was prepared to do jumping jacks or headstands or anything else that might provide an answer to my question.

I went with her to the seminar and listened with interest as Renu spoke about misconceptions about astrology and misuse of this information, which was all about exploration, getting to know the forces of nature set in motion when we take our first breath, energy that surrounds us and marks our souls. She challenged us to consider what we wanted to learn from this life. I couldn't buy into everything she was saying, but for some purely instinctual reason, I liked her. I wanted to hear more.

Valeria had forgotten to tell me that everyone was supposed to send their name, birth date, and other information in advance so Renu could prepare their charts, and we were all supposed to be following along, chart in hand, as she spoke. I was missing this vital piece of the presentation. During the first break, I went over to Renu and asked her if there was any way I could still participate.

"Of course," she said and handily whipped up the intricate chart with a computer program. (A program for ancient wisdom. This is the world we live in now.)

She skimmed the baffling rows and boxes filled with impossibly tiny print, calculations, and algorithms.

"You are very water," she said. "That can be a puddle or a river."

Her brow furrowed. "You're having a hard time. We should talk."

Right, I thought dryly, but the light touch of her hand on my shoulder felt genuine.

She told me I was going through *Sade Sati*, and I tried to keep up as she told me in her animated way about *ketu dasha*, intergenerational molecular memories, and all sorts of ideas that sounded like complete outer-spacey nutball stuff, but every once in a while there was a kernel of undeniable wisdom in it.

"You're in pain," she said. "You've experienced a great loss."

"My grandmother." I couldn't say any more than that. My throat felt tight. *A great loss.* The words were so small, and the reality so profound I started crying.

"*Sade Sati* is more emotional than physical," she said. "It's the Etch A Sketch being shaken so we can wipe clean every thirty years all the dark memories we're carrying in our consciousness. And it's not all bad. It can be good. Pressure comes from all sides, and it's like squeezing a lemon. Whatever is in there is going to come out. And this is good. Trauma surfaces to be healed."

I took all this in, trying to hang on to those moments that resonated. I loved her pragmatic humor—the way she described Saturn as "an old grumpy grandpa" and accepted without judgment every person's doubt or faith. There was no lightning bolt of truth here, no epiphany that would change the world or my mind, but I'll tell you what did click into place—if not in that moment, then very soon after. Nothing the doctors were telling me resonated for me any more than the concept of *ketu dasha*. The medical doctors I'd been seeing would probably have rolled their eyes at the idea that my body and soul were off on separate misadventures, but when they told me there was nothing wrong with me, they were asking me to accept on faith something I knew was untrue. At least Renu was listening to me and acknowledging that something was wrong.

I arranged to meet with her at her home in North Austin. Sitting in her office, I felt calm and welcome. There was none of the adversarial loin-girding I felt going into an appointment where I knew I'd have to plead for a few minutes' attention or insist on being heard. Renu, serene and beautiful in her flowy orange blouse and white palazzo pants, was easy to sit with. The air felt open and free of anxiety. Confiding in her felt natural.

As Renu and I continued to meet for long, wide-ranging conversations, I became more and more fascinated, by the subject matter and by Renu herself. Renu comes from a well-respected Indian family. Her father was a UN ambassador, so she lived in Switzerland for a time. She married a man who came from royalty, but his family refused to accept her and disinherited him. You can tell when you talk with her that she grew up with a wealth of opportunities for travel and education, but there's nothing ostentatious or entitled about her. Humble and wise, she listens more than she talks, and when she does talk, her voice has a calming rhythm and melody.

I wanted to learn more about the philosophy of Vedic healing, so I organized a class and invited her to come and teach me and a few friends. Several of my friends were as fascinated as I was, but having been raised in a very different belief system, most of us remained skeptical. After the class, I asked Renu, "What do you call someone who doesn't believe in any of this stuff?"

"My husband," she laughed.

Renu's guru is known all over the world as Amma, the Hugging Saint, famous for her dedication to helping the poor and for her darshan—the motherly hug she gives to thousands of people who come to her. Amma is, in essence, the Hindu version of Mother Teresa. The ideology she passed along to Renu is a progressive understanding of ancient wisdom, applied with a utilitarian compassion. Eduardo and I went with Renu to meet Amma in Santa Fe. When Renu saw my suitcase full of black pants, jeans, and colorful tunic blouses, she laughed and said, "We must wear white."

We went to buy some Indian clothes, and as we shopped, she told me more about Amma's teachings.

"She acknowledges the poetic justice of karma," said Renu, "but she refuses to allow karma to be used as an excuse for inaction. If one person's karma means suffering, then another person's dharma must be helping."

"How does one find that helper person?" I asked.

"Karma."

Later that day, waiting for our turn to speak with Amma and receive that famous hug, I clutched a photograph of my children in my hand. I was desperate for any miracle, any level of blessing. The truth is, I was terrified by what was happening to me. I wanted to beg her, *Please, help me. I think I'm dying.* But when I knelt in front of her, Eduardo kneeling beside me, I said, "Please . . . bless my family. I want to be with my children."

Amma gave me an apple and said something about my sweetness. Her wisdom and empathy were evident, and I was astonished at the energy of this elderly lady—to sit there hour after hour, listening, taking in the sorrows of others and responding with pristinely calm compassion.

"Amma tells us that love expressed is compassion," Renu told me on the way home. "Compassion means embracing the sorrow of another as if it's our own."

I ate the apple Amma had given me, trying to feel some aspect of its sweetness reflected in myself, but that great loss Renu had sensed in me—though I had immediately connected that word to the loss of my grandmother—was in fact the loss of myself. This physical malaise that made my head pound and my body ache was robbing me of my spirit.

Health is inclusive. For better or worse, body and soul are stuck with each other. This shouldn't come as such a surprise to us. Separation of body and soul is the very definition of death! How do we not compute that life means bringing the body and soul into harmony? Eat an apple. Eat a bottle of blue pills. I began to wonder: What difference does one make without the other?

five

Here's a little Endocrinology 101: the organs and glands in your endocrine system, most notably the "trinity"—the pituitary master gland in your brain and two adrenal glands perched atop your kidneys—regulate hormones that control vital functions like blood pressure, heart rate, metabolism, growth, fertility, and a host of other bodily functions we never even think about until they go wrong. At this very moment, there are up to forty different hormones zooming through your blood vessels, carrying critical messages to your brain, heart, lungs, muscles, skin—every part of you that lives, breathes, thinks, feels, and grows. The message is received, a hormonal response is sent back, and the conversation goes on. *Okay, that's enough of that, thank you, but we need a little more of this . . .*

Your brilliant body is engineered to maintain, protect, and heal itself in a million big and small ways using hormones that integrate body, mind, and emotion. PMS is one perfect example. Women are shamed into thinking that this wave of hormones and the moodiness that comes with PMS is a weakness, but in fact, it's a powerful healing mechanism. Studies have shown that "reflex tears" prompted by slicing an onion or getting poked in the eye are 98 percent water, while tears prompted by emotion are filled with excess hormones and stress-induced toxins. Masking, medicating, and stuffing emotion prevents the body from healing itself, so the body releases more hormones, telling the brain, *Help me out here. Make this girl cry.* So the mind goes where it needs to go in order to produce the necessary level of emotion until the body cries, excreting toxins, and then the brain rewards Team Weepy with a comforting fizz of endorphins. And that's why you feel better after you've had a good cry. Training ourselves not to cry is, quite literally, poisonous.

On a purely mechanical level, it is impossible to separate the well-being of the body from the well-being of the mind and spirit. Endocrinology, as I understand it, is the science of harmonizing the hormones that regulate the body, brain, and spirit, and that overall harmony is essential to a person's well-being on every level.

My sister's intense situation—thyroid cancer amid the hormonal rodeo of pregnancy—required a vigilant endocrinologist. We were grateful to find Dr. Thomas Blevins. He helped guide her through the whole ordeal and kept a watchful eye on her, especially during that first year after the baby was born and Roby's body was readjusting to its new circumstances.

In spring 2013, a year after my sister's cancer diagnosis, I drove her to a follow-up appointment at Dr. Blevins's office in Austin. As I sat with her in the waiting room, the overhead lights created a drum roll in my temples. I closed my eyes, twisting a heavy silver ring on my right hand, working it until my finger was red and swollen. The idea of getting the weight of that ring off my finger took root in my mind and crept like ivy until it was all I could think about. *Get it off. Get it off. Why won't it come off?* I finally managed to rake it over my raw knuckle, and my mind instantly fixed on the weight of my earrings. And my bracelet. So I clawed those off as well.

The receptionist called Roby's name. I shoved the silver accessories into my purse and followed my sister to the hallway, where the nurse took all the usual vitals: weight, height, blood pressure, and temp. In the exam room, we started chatting cheerfully about where we might go to lunch after the appointment since Mami was watching our babies. It was good to see Roby happy and healed, no longer feeling fragile. I squeezed her hand and took the chair in the corner. A painting of longhorn cattle loomed over us, munching prairie grass, waiting in silence with us.

I studied a poster that detailed the warning signs for thyroid trouble. On the desk below it was a little wooden model labeled *Right Kidney and Adrenal Gland.* The kidney was mounted on a wooden dowel like a mutant Mr. Potato Head, topped with a spongy, pointed cap—like the jaunty little cap Peter Pan wears in the animated movie—and it occurs to me now that I didn't even wonder, *Gosh, what do you suppose that silly little cap is for?* (The answer is, *Everything!*)

There was a soft knock on the door before Dr. Blevins breezed in, exactly on time, tall and lanky with a ready smile and easy manner.

"Hello, Roby," he said, gripping her hand between his. "How's the baby?"

"Wonderful," she replied. "Dr. Blevins, this is my sister, Lorena."

"Good to meet you, Lorena."

I felt him studying me as I reached out to accept his warm handshake. Pleasant small talk continued as Dr. Blevins palpated my sister's scarred neck where the thyroid had been. She sat up straight, and he stood behind her, moving his hands around her neck, tracing the line of her collarbone with his index finger. A nurse wheeled in a sonogram machine, and I closed my eyes, listening to the faint hum and quiet cross talk. When the procedure was finished, Dr. Blevins flipped open a thick file folder.

"Let's go over these test results. Potassium levels . . . triiodothy-ronine . . . T3 . . . T4 . . ."

As the words and numbers sounded like a stream of random sounds and syllables, we sat there nodding as if it made sense. We assumed he knew what he was talking about, and that's what mattered. I was startled when he closed the folder and turned to me.

"Lorena," he said, "given your sister's history, I think it would be wise to check your thyroid as well."

"Okay . . ."

My hand went to my neck. Over the past year or so, I'd gotten used to a vague puffiness that had settled there. My collarbone wasn't as sharply defined as it used to be. Dr. Blevins returned his attention to Roby, but before we left his office, he handed me some paperwork.

I scheduled blood tests for later that week and returned to Dr. Blevins's office to hear the results. As I followed the nurse down the hall, stood on the scale, and offered my arm for the blood pressure cuff, I steeled myself for the familiar results. *Nothing to see here. Move along, folks.* I prepared myself for that familiar gut-punched feeling I had every time another doctor told me, "Everything's fine." The longhorn cattle munched on the wall, comfortably assured that my misery was all in my imagination.

Dr. Blevins came in, and we exchanged pleasantries. He went into that incomprehensible stream of syllables and numbers, and I nodded, listening for something that made sense.

"Hm." He paused. "Hypokalemia. Very low potassium levels."

"What does that mean?"

"Could mean a number of different things." He considered it for a moment and then reached for the prescription pad. "This medication is prescription-grade potassium—a heavy dose. Make sure you follow the directions."

I took the powerful medicine, waiting for something to change, but when I returned to follow up with Dr. Blevins, he said, "It's not working. Let's get a CT scan."

"I've already had brain scans," I said, but he shook his head.

"We need to look at the adrenal glands. Those are in your abdomen."

Okay. Whatever works, I figured. I appreciated his willingness to explore beyond the obvious. I headed home to consult Dr. Google about the role of the adrenal glands.

Lying in the CT scan machine, my head buzzed like a beehive, but I allowed myself to hope for some kind of answer, even if it was something that scared me. Having seen Dr. Blevins a few times now, I'd come to trust him. I loved his manner, the way he asked and remembered the names of my children, and the fact that he followed up with me with test results and next steps. Even so, I was surprised to see his number on my cell a few days later. It was after eight at night. I was on my way home from a fund raiser at my kids' school.

"Hello, Dr. Blevins." I pulled over to the shoulder of the road, emergency blinkers ticking in the falling dusk.

"Hi, Lorena. I need to speak with you about your CT scan. Is this a good time?"

"Um . . . sure. What is it?"

"There's a 1.4-centimeter tumor on your adrenal gland."

My long, private struggle distilled to crystal clarity. The answer. All my questions collapsed into the black hole of an answer the size of a lima bean.

"Is it cancer?" I asked.

"Adrenal tumors are rarely malignant," he said, "but they can cause a lot of trouble. We can tell from your potassium and magnesium levels that this tumor is active, so we need to see to it right away. Call my office tomorrow for an appointment. I can refer you to a good surgeon."

"Okay. Yes."

"See you soon, Lorena. Don't worry. We'll get it taken care of."

"Thank you," I said. "Thank you for calling."

I almost laughed. Almost cried. After all this, could it be that simple? *We'll get it taken care of.* Just a little snip, a few stitches, and this whole nightmare would be over. I was scared by the ominous words—*tumor, surgery, hospital*—of course, these are scary words, but my concern for the coming procedure was nothing compared to the nagging fear I'd been living with. The bad thing you know about is never as terrifying as the bad thing in your imagination.

I turned off the blinkers and headed home, feeling like I was breathing for the first time in twenty months. Soon I would be myself again—the caregiver instead of the one who needs to be taken care of.

When I was twelve, I used to volunteer at a nursing home—a state asylum-type facility, not some fancy retirement home. Every Saturday my parents would drop me off at the nursing home where I spent the day doing crafts, aiding in personal hygiene, and keeping company with the elderly and infirm people who needed full-time care. I brought them meals and coffee, changed adult diapers, listened to their stories, and helped them make little clay picture frames and papier-mâché boxes for their treasures.

I came to care about the elderly people who shuffled from room to room, expending so much effort at such a slow pace. It was like helping giant turtles cross the freeway. The world kept whirling around these people, and they couldn't keep up with it anymore, so they sat still with their rich histories on the walls of their rooms, and I sat with them. I'm not sure why I felt such a deep affinity for these mostly forgotten souls. They were someone else's great-grandparents, but they needed to feel loved, and I loved feeling needed.

Caregiving is a privilege that feeds the soul and grows the heart, and if we're to be totally honest, there's a kernel of selfishness in it. It feels good to give because it requires you to recognize the bounty you have. It's empowering. You're in control, the strong one. Receiving care, on the other hand, requires humility and patience and a lot of other things we'd all rather not think about. I had not learned this yet, because I'd been a caregiver all my life. I'm not saying I never needed help, but when I did need help, I paid for it or I helped the other person in return. I always knew that this was an equal exchange of goods and services. I wasn't indebted to anyone. My pride was intact, and all things were even.

My instinct to give care has always been strong and immediate when it came to other people. Being my own caregiver was a conscious decision I had to grow into. Being a caregiver to yourself means listening to and believing yourself, opening the same open heart you would open to a loved one. It means fighting for answers, the same way you would advocate for your child. It means taking ownership of whatever you're experiencing, weighing the advice and opinions of others, but never ignoring your own gut feeling. If you don't feel right, don't let anyone tell you, "There's nothing wrong." Understand that what they're actually saying is, "I don't know what's wrong, and not knowing scares me, so I'm going to pretend it's nothing." It does you no good to pretend along with them. You can't afford to be afraid. You, as your own caregiver, must be brave and continue your search for the truth.

On my way home that night, eager to share the diagnosis and Dr. Blevins's reassuring words with Eduardo, I was experiencing a monsoon of mixed emotions, but overall, I felt hopeful. I fully anticipated a smooth return to good health and my old self. I had no idea what it would feel like when I was forced to swallow my pride and accept what was about to happen to me. The hard lessons I'd already learned—about being my own caregiver and about the fallibility of doctors—would become more important than I could imagine.

Back in Dr. Blevins's office a few days later, I took in the flood of information. In addition to the damage it had already wreaked on my general health, the aldosterone-producing adenoma was putting me at risk for hypertension, heart attack, and stroke. It was a relief to finally have a name for this thing that had been stealing my life from me, but alarming to know how much worse it might have been. I didn't flinch at the idea of having the entire adrenal gland removed. We're born with two, so I'd still have a functional adrenal gland with which I could recover and continue my life.

Dr. Blevins suggested two well-respected surgeons. One was Dr. Humano. When Dr. Blevins mentioned his name, I said, "Oh, I know Dr. Humano. He did my hernia repair surgery after my son, Eddie, was born."

"And that went well?"

"Yes, very well," I said. "I liked him."

Dr. Humano had impressed me with his kindness and professionalism. He had a terrific bedside manner, built a relationship with us, and followed up. In that moment, I trusted Dr. Humano with my body, and he seemed to understand that it was a sacred trust.

"He's an excellent surgeon," said Dr. Blevins. "If you feel good about it, I'd definitely recommend that we have him do the procedure."

So it was settled. And I did feel good about it. I wouldn't be trusting this vital moment to a stranger. Dr. Humano, a caregiver I trusted, would be there to help me.

Six

Not much had changed at Dr. Humano's office since I was there for my last follow-up appointment after the hernia surgery: sliding glass doors in the lobby and all the usual furnishings in the waiting room. When the receptionist called my name, my stomach tightened. *Here we go.* I was anxious to get past the pain and focus on healing. I followed her down the hall—weight, height, vitals—and waited in the exam room for Dr. Humano.

He hadn't changed much, either. Dr. Humano is tall and lanky with a gentle voice, keen eyes, and a long, crooked nose. His hands are good hands for a surgeon, elegant and perfectly manicured. His demeanor is respectful and caring, starting with the way he knocks lightly on the door before opening it. As he conducts his examination, he talks you through it, asking for permission before proceeding. "I'm going to open the robe. Is that okay?" He listens with all the right body language, leaning forward, intent on what you're saying.

Everything about his bedside manner is appropriate and authoritative, and something about that paternal air made me want to be a good patient. I felt compelled to please him, to say the right things and be brave. This wasn't just the usual impulse to please, like wanting the other moms to like you or keeping up your cocktail party game face. This was a strong feeling that my cheerful cooperation was important to the outcome of my surgery.

Dr. Humano didn't do anything in particular to make me think this. He didn't have to. We're both products of a system in which a tall white male doctor and a woman patient cross paths in a well-choreographed pattern. Neither of us has to do or say anything to create that unspoken dynamic. No one does. It just is what it is. If you don't actively disrupt it, it continues, and the last thing I wanted to do in that moment was disrupt things. I wanted things to go smoothly. I wanted to be well taken care of.

We chatted briefly about my family, how Eddie—who was a newborn baby last time Dr. Humano saw me—was a rambunctious toddler now. Then Dr. Humano flipped open my file.

"I've reviewed your scans and the test results," he said. "Your blood pressure is up, which is not surprising. We'll give you something for that."

We never discussed the possibility of a partial adrenalectomy. He was recommending a complete unilateral adrenalectomy, meaning that he would remove the entire gland and leave the other gland intact.

"We should be able to do a laparoscopic adrenalectomy," he said. "Very small incisions. Very short recovery. You'll be in and out within a few hours."

"I don't even stay overnight?"

"Barring any unforeseen problems, you'll be able to go home that same day and be back to normal activities within a week."

"What about travel? Eduardo and I are planning a big family trip in a few weeks."

He shrugged his angular shoulders. "Shouldn't be a problem."

"Okay. Great," I said. "That's wonderful. How soon can you do the surgery? I want to do it now. As soon as possible."

I didn't want to sound like I was begging—*Fix it! Fix it now!*—but for so long I'd been feeling like I was at the end of my rope. Now that a solution was within reach, I couldn't sit here pretending to be nonchalant about it.

"I'll check my schedule," he said.

I walked with him to the front desk where his assistant pulled up his schedule and said, "Looks like the first available date is next week."

"Perfect," I said.

I went home feeling hopeful and reassured. In that morning, out that afternoon. I couldn't believe it was that simple.

And, of course, it wasn't.

Seven

Eduardo and I had been planning a once-in-a-lifetime family reunion: a three-generation visit to a lovely historic home where my whole family was to stay together, immersed in the richness and culture of Mexico, riding bicycles, playing games, and visiting galleries and museums. My kids adore the process of creating this kind of educational summer vacation and dove into the research, watching historical videos and movies to set the background. Papi, who loves to be the fun grandpa, planned to hang swings from the tree branches and arrange scooters and other activities for the children.

Sitting at my kitchen table, sipping Topo Chico and nibbling crackers, I smiled and tried to focus on plans for the adventure. Mami's eyes were full of joy and anticipation that should have been contagious, but I felt numb and detached.

"It'll be so much fun," she said. "And the art, Lorena—I know this is just what you need to get your energy back."

My mother's voice came and went, raising images of trees, flowers, and children playing, but a cocoon of dead air enveloped me. I wanted to feel joy. Something was stopping me.

"Lorena? Are you listening to me?"

"Yes, but I can't think about that right now. I have this surgery coming up."

"You'll be fine," she said. "You're in good hands with Dr. Humano. You'll be back on your feet in no time."

"I know, but I don't want to wait. I'm so ready to get this over with. I'm so done with feeling rotten." I rested my head in my hands, trying to organize my thoughts. "You all should go ahead as planned. Take the kids. Please. I'll get the surgery done and join you as soon as I can."

"Lorena! No. I'm not leaving you here to go through the surgery all alone."

"I won't be alone, Mami, and I can't put it off. Don't change your plans for me."

"Don't be ridiculous. Your family should be with you. Or maybe your father and Eduardo should go with the children. I'll stay here with you."

Eduardo was as surprised as my mother was, and as adamant that he should be here with me, but I was determined to handle this myself without disrupting the family adventure. Mami had devoted a lot of time and energy to planning it, the kids were over the moon with excitement, and all that aside, I wanted to take charge of the situation myself. Fighting for this diagnosis, I'd felt like I had no control over the situation. Now I wanted to be in the driver's seat. With the firm diagnosis on my chart, I had research I could focus on and decisions I could make. It felt good to finally take charge and move forward. I was ready.

"And I won't be alone," I assured Mami. "I'll have family with me."

I'd already arranged everything. Roby, and Eduardo's parents, Tía Paty and Tío Ricardo, would be there for me when I woke up.

I knew it was hard for my parents to leave, but the best thing they could do for me in that moment was make sure my kids were safe and happy so I could focus on myself for a few days. This was the best way for everyone, I was certain, but that didn't make it easy, and ultimately, Eduardo insisted that he would fly back for the surgery after he got the children settled with Mami and Papi at their home-away-from-home.

My family left for vacation without me. Tía Paty and Tío Ricardo took me out to an early dinner. I knew exactly what time I should stop eating and drinking. I went home and sorted through all the paperwork one more time: insurance forms, presurgery instructions, and hospital admittance. As the time ticked by, I drank as much water as I could stomach. I didn't want to get dehydrated. As I read through all the papers again and organized them in a file folder, I kept one eye on the clock.

One more hour to drink water.

Half an hour left to drink water.

Five minutes left to drink water.

I laid out everything I would need. Loose cotton pants, comfy shirt, socks and slip-on shoes, so I'd have something easy to go home in. A shawl to wrap around my shoulders because they always keep it cool in the recovery room. Lip balm and hand lotion for the dry Texas summer air. A book to distract me while I waited for the anesthesiologist's meds to kick in. I packed each item into my bag, mentally rehearsing the day surgery routine: get there, gown up, meet each member of the surgical team when they stop by, someone starts the IV, and then it's sleep, snip, stitch, and then you wake up wondering what time it is. After a few hours of ice chips and TV in the recovery room, you force yourself out of bed to use the bathroom, and (ideally) head home in time for a groggy dinner of soup and crackers.

Eduardo called me to report that the kids were having a blast and he was on his way to the airport.

"I should be landing right about the time they take you back for surgery," he said. "I'll be there when you wake up."

"I'm glad you're coming," I confessed. "When you get here, please pay attention and take good notes. I might be feeling woozy afterward, and I want to make sure I get all the information."

I made myself go to bed early, but I lay awake, periodically looking at my phone, calculating and recalculating how much sleep I would get if I could will myself to drift off *right now*.

Now? Six hours.

Okay, now? Five hours.

How about now? Three hours and forty-five minutes.

Sleep finally found me, but my alarm went off after what seemed like only a few minutes. It was summertime now, so the early sunrise washed the sky with watercolor pink and purple. I allowed myself to hit the snooze button—only once—and lay there listening to the empty house, missing everyone more than I expected I would.

Before I stepped into the shower, I visited the little meditation corner in my closet, a small sacred space I had created for thought and gratitude. On top of the shoe cupboard was a photograph of Eduardo and me, young and in love, and a picture of my parents, laughing and windblown on the beach. Beside a cairn of stones and rose quartz, there was a painting of Jesus in a small rococo gold frame. Two small votives—Italian ceramic filled with seeds—held my offerings to motherhood and fertility, and next to them, I'd set Paty's worn ballet slipper and a note in Lore's preschool scrawl:

Mom you are the bist.

I breathed in the memories and love, breathed out weariness and presurgery jitters. *Breathe in. Breathe out. Today is a good day. Today I turn the corner and become myself again.*

When I stepped out of the shower, I heard voices downstairs. It was Tía Paty and Tío Ricardo. Good. Everything going according to plan. I smelled breakfast cooking and wished I could eat, but I was following instructions to the letter, determined to have this day go off without a hitch. I pulled on baggy clothes and scooped my hair into a messy bun.

On my way down the wide stone stairway, I paused at a little alcove where I had installed large pieces of quartz. I have quartz, crystals, and geodes, some the size of an egg, some as big as cinder blocks, stationed throughout my home. They make me think of my grandmother. I like to think of them as ancient guardians—patron saints in my own private theology—and I've assigned each one a different task. Protect Eduardo's study. Watch over the game room. One particular quartz obelisk in the stairway alcove was charged with safeguarding our good health. I held it between my hands for a moment.

Breathe in. Breathe out.

When Tía Paty saw me, she smiled and set a reassuring hand on my shoulder. "How are you?"

"Good," I said. "Ready to do this."

Roby arrived and took me into a tight hug. She seemed quiet, and I noticed how she sat with her hand on her midsection.

"Are you all right?" I asked.

"I don't know. My stomach is a little off."

She was back on her feet, feeling strong and well, but she was still coping with the emotional aftermath of cancer. It's possible that she was feeling some anxiety about going back to the hospital, but she didn't mention it or complain about not feeling well. She was as determined to be there for me as I was to be there for her.

"Eduardo called last night," I said. "Sounds like the kids are having a blast."

"I'm sure they are," she laughed.

"I can't wait to be there with them."

"Soon," said Tía Paty, and she squeezed my shoulder again. "Shall we get going?"

No one had to ask me twice. I was the first one to the car, getting anxious when I was still waiting for everyone else a few minutes later.

"Roby's not feeling well," she said. "I tried to tell her she should stay here, but she insisted on being with you."

"Oh, no. Is she okay?"

"She'll be fine. Look, here she comes."

Roby climbed in with a smile. "Good to go."

I nodded and closed my eyes, willing away the butterflies in my own stomach. It was comforting to pull into the breezeway behind the hospital—the first of many omens telling me I was in the right place. Last time I came out of those doors, I had a new baby in my arms. As I searched for signs that all would be well, the joy of that moment eclipsed any fears I had about going inside.

The hospital staff moved everything along like a well-maintained machine. I handed off the paperwork I'd prepared the night before and worked through the fresh paperwork required to get started. The nurse placed a plastic band around my wrist, and every time someone had me sign something or step on the scale or offer my arm for the blood pressure cuff, they looked at my red latex-allergy bracelet and cross-referenced the name and number on my chart. So much checking and double-checking. It was very reassuring.

Behind a curtain in the pre-op area, I got into my hospital gown and pulled on a blue robe. The nurse tied my hair back and covered it with a hairnet.

"I have thin veins," I told her as she searched for a spot to start the IV. "Sometimes it takes a few tries."

"We'll see," she said, rising to the challenge, but it took her three pokes with a pediatric needle to get the line going.

Once I was in bed, Tía Paty and Roby were allowed to come in and sit with me. Tío Ricardo stayed in the waiting room, watching for Eduardo. Trying to keep the mood light, we all engaged in a conversation about empanada recipes. Tía Paty patted Roby's hand and complimented the beautiful bracelet Roby was wearing.

"Definitely prettier than mine," I said, holding out my arm with the plastic band.

Roby laughed and said, "Yours is probably more expensive."

We were glad to go on like this, chatting about everything and nothing, until the anesthesiologist came in. He greeted me with a pleasant handshake, checked the IV, and went directly to the list of standard questions on his clipboard.

"Any allergies?"

"Latex," I said. "And sulfas."

"Got it. Any alcohol consumed in the past week?"

"No."

"Drugs or tobacco products?"

"No."

"Wait . . ." He flipped back a page or two on the clipboard, doing a double take. "Lorena?"

"Oh . . . Tim!" I hadn't realized the anesthesiologist was my neighbor. We both laughed when we recognized each other in our surgical garb, as if we were at a costume party. It's funny how you don't always recognize someone out of context, isn't it? But for me, at the time, this felt like another good omen.

"This is just something to help you relax." He produced a syringe and pushed the contents into the IV. "See you in the OR."

The curtain scraped open. A nurse helped me onto a gurney, and after quick hugs from my loved ones, an orderly wheeled me down the hall. I shivered under the cold sheets. Fluorescent lights skimmed by like the windows of a passing train. The nurse positioned the gurney at the center of the OR and asked, "How are you doing?"

"I'm good."

Dr. Humano arrived, bringing that air of fatherly authority with him. His confidence was comforting.

"Good morning, Lorena," he said. "How are you doing?"

"I'm good. I'm ready."

"Good." He surveyed the instruments laid out on the table and consulted the paperwork clipped to my chart. "So, we are taking out the left adrenal gland today."

"Yes."

"Lorena," said Tim, "I'm going to give you a cocktail that will make you feel a bit groggy, okay?"

"Okay. Thank you." I waited, wanting to feel myself slipping under. "I'm not feeling anything yet. Should I be feeling something?"

"It'll come," he said.

I felt a little silly for asking. *Breathe in. Breathe out.*

I lay in the operating theater, visualizing a blanket of white light.

"How are we doing, Lorena?"

I opened my eyes and saw Dr. Humano's warm, smiling eyes.

"Uh-huh . . ." I said. And then I was gone.

According to my medical records:

The patient was taken to operating room 17 and placed supine. General endotracheal anesthesia was established uneventfully.

The patient was then turned in modified partial left lateral position with kidney rest elevated to widen the distance between the left costal margin and the left hip. Beanbag for stabilization. SCDs had been applied.

A Foley catheter was not required . . . Procedure well tolerated, no complications.

Sponge, instrument, and needle counts correct.

Returned supine, extubated in the operating room, brought to recovery in good condition.

When I look at Dr. Humano's concise description of the uncomplicated procedure that forever complicated my life, I feel his unshakable confidence. It was a routine surgery, something he'd probably done hundreds of times before. But reading over these notes, which I have now done hundreds if not thousands of times, I find it interesting that the grammar is in the passive voice: *This was done.* Never the active voice: *I did this.*

Generic items are moved around like props on a stage: the beanbag, the hip, the patient. There's nothing in those notes that speaks to the necessary violence of surgery. People resist that word in this context. It took me years to come to terms with it myself because I thought *violence* requires a *victim,* and I didn't want to think of myself that way. When I say that surgery is violent, I'm not talking about harmful results or cruel intentions; I'm talking about trauma to the body that must be honored before it can be healed. Surgery is invasive, even when it goes the way it's supposed to. We have to give our bodies credit for that and allow the time and patience required for healing.

But I doubt any surgeon wants to think of his craft in terms of *violence* or *trauma.* The intention is to fix whatever is broken, so that's the surgeon's focus. Perhaps it's too painful to think of it any other way. Looking back on those surgical notes, Dr. Humano's confidence sounds more like disconnection to me. There's a guard up. But that is my inexpert reading, Eduardo reminds me, so I try not to read too much into it. It is what it is. Everyone in their proper place. I suppose if a surgeon were to allow any crack in that cinder block wall that surrounds his comfort zone, the miasma of insecurity might seep in. If the body placed supine on the gurney was a woman, a mother, a wife, a human being, an artist, exposed and utterly vulnerable—that might be unnerving, and we all want a surgeon with nerves of titanium. Better to have everyone on both sides of the scalpel keep their masks in place, remain anonymous. Passive. In the correct context.

For the patient, no such disconnect is possible. It's stunning to think of how vulnerable your body is in the surgical theater: naked, dormant, exposed. Laparoscopic surgery is the least invasive procedure possible, and I was glad for that. Dr. Humano made five small incisions in the immediate vicinity of my belly button: two for his instruments, two for his assistant's instruments, and one for the camera. I don't think he actually saw the inside of me with his own eyes; he watched the scenery go by on a computer screen, guiding the instruments with the practiced moves of a professional *World of Warcraft* gamer. All very technical. Very precise. He located the adrenal gland—a five-gram lump of tissue, that little Peter Pan hat—snipped it free from the kidney, and sucked it out through a narrow cannula.

I'm curious to know how that felt to him. Was there a frisson of satisfaction, like that small thrill you feel when you pop bubble wrap? *Floop!* Up the cannula it went. When he snapped off his gloves, his hands were clean. I'm curious to know what he was thinking. Did he glance at the time? Had he mentally moved on to the next task already? Did another body lay waiting, naked and dormant, in the next room?

eight

I've seen a sculpture by Damien Hirst, who is known for his extravagant, evocative, and sometimes playful use of the human skull. *The Skull (Exploded): The Dream Is Dead* captures precisely what it feels like to have a migraine. An aching jaw drops away from jagged cheekbone fragments. The forehead hovers above the void where a face should be, held up by slender titanium rods, and the crown flies apart in shards, leaving only a glimpse of what a human head should look like.

That was me as I emerged from the fog of anesthesia with an intense headache and the strange sensation of cold air dragging at my feet like a riptide. This was not my first migraine. I'd been having them since I was a girl—since we moved from Monterrey to Mexico City, to be exact—but this was not the usual migraine. This was something with a life of its own.

My fingers were curled around the square metal post that supported the bedside table. I wanted to let go, but I couldn't. I looked at my hand, and it was like looking at the hooked claws of a dead bird. The sheets felt as chalky and stiff as raw drywall. A shadow moved toward the head of the bed, shades of vein blue and fog white. A nurse. I was in the hospital. I tried to speak to her, but my mouth felt starched and dry.

"Lorena? Lorena, can you talk to me? How are you feeling?"

She rubbed my arm briskly. My body felt like shattered plaster.

"Sleepy," I managed. "My head hurts."

When she moved the bed to a sitting-up position, the pressure in my skull became a vise that gripped my temples and made my eyes feel too big for their sockets. I was afraid to move.

"Do you need to use the bathroom, Lorena? Let's try to get you up. We can't let you go home until you use the bathroom."

I did need to pee, but I couldn't get up. And I couldn't imagine what she was talking about. Go home? Like this?

"I can't. Please." My voice sounded thready and weak. "Don't send me home."

"We won't send you till you're ready," she said. "Let's see how you do in recovery."

The transition from bed to wheelchair was a monstrous effort that left me trembling with exhaustion. As she wheeled me to the recovery room, I closed my eyes, nauseated by the carousel motion of the doors and lights and people going by. I became aware of myself in fragments, puzzle pieces I couldn't seem to reassemble. My feet were numb clubs. Long muscles in my legs twitched and spasmed. My neck and shoulders felt tightly wired above my hammering chest. My head was an exploding star. In the middle of me, there was . . . nothing. An unnerving void separated the upper and lower parts of me, the way a magician's assistant is separated after she's been sawed in two. The only thing holding me together was a cocoon of dull agony.

"Here we are."

The wheelchair lurched to a halt. The nurse spoke quietly with someone else. Another nurse, maybe. Their voices rose and fell between the blood rushing in my ears.

". . . here for another hour . . . see how she feels . . ."

". . . keep her overnight if . . . be best for her to stay . . ."

Arms tentacled around me, lifting me into another bed. Strange arms. I wanted my sister.

"Roby?"

"She wasn't well, sweetie." Tía Paty spoke close to my ear. "We had to take her home. How are you?"

I couldn't form thoughts, couldn't find words, but I felt Eduardo take my hand, and I let myself be tethered to that for a while.

"*Mi amor*, what happened?"

"It went perfectly," he said.

"But . . . what was . . . did he say . . . anything?"

"He said it went perfectly. You're going to be fine." I could hear the relief in his voice. "It's over, *mi amorcito*. It's done."

"I'm thirsty."

"No water yet." The nurse hovered nearby again, doing something with the IV. "Try some ice chips."

She slipped a chunk of ice into my mouth. It made my teeth feel like broken glass, but I was grateful for the cool trickle of moisture in my throat. I lay for a long time, trembling and sweating. When I closed my eyes, I could feel the room reeling around me. When I opened my eyes, the fluorescent lights became arrows and knives. Usually, when I have a migraine, I retreat to my room and just unplug from all the light and noise. Eventually, I sink into blackness and sleep it off. This migraine kept me twisting, wanting to crawl out of my skin. The clanging in my ears wouldn't let me sleep. For the rest of the day, I lay suspended between consciousness and unconsciousness, and nightmares waited for me either way.

Eduardo and his parents came and went quietly, fetching each other coffee, roaming from hallway to waiting room to cafeteria and back again. Tía Paty is a German lady who keeps calm wits about her in every situation. Tío Ricardo hates hospitals, but he loves me and would not have been anywhere else but here. They were vigilant about my care and protective about my modesty. They brought a calm, sensible presence to the room, and I was grateful.

Every two hours, a nurse came to check my vitals. Every four hours, she gave me something for the pain. They drew blood, pricking again and again, searching for the tricky veins. I clutched a remote control in my hand. I was supposed to get some kind of medication for the pain every time I pushed the button. It was supposed to make me feel like I was in control of it. Beside the bed, there was a poster with numbers 1 to 10 beneath shouty caps:

PAIN ASSESSMENT TOOL

Below the numbered scale was a row of cartoon faces meant to demonstrate what your pain was supposed to look like. As if my pain and your pain are interchangeable. As if either of our pain looks like a constipated emoji.

0 was a verdant green smile: *No Pain*

1 to 3 was an uncomfortable chartreuse: *Mild*

4 to 6 was a pasty amber grimace: *Moderate*

7 to 9 was an alarming orange frown: *Severe*

10 was a bawling red nevus: *Worst Pain Possible*

As if anyone knows what sort of pain is the worst possible for someone else. Pain is personal. It's unique. I understand the clinical need to quantify it, but the first time I had a migraine, I would have described it as the worst pain possible, and now here I was, proving that assumption wrong. Is *this* pain the "worst pain possible"? I would hope to God that it is! But who knows?

"How is the pain?" The nurse pointed at the center of the spectrum, where she figured I should be. "About a five?"

"Nine," I said, and I could tell from her expression that this was the wrong answer. I insisted, "It's not a ten, but it is a nine."

"Okay . . ." she said, tapping her pen on her chin.

It was clear in her expression that I had not given the right answer. I was not being a good patient. I was not doing pain right.

"Maybe . . . a six?" I said, and this seemed to please her. She wrote it down on my chart and patted my shoulder. I longed for my mother. She always says I have a very high pain threshold. She would have known that nine means nine. The nurse was happier with the lie, but the lie made me feel even more isolated and broken.

I dozed, and when I woke up, I did feel somewhat better. The migraine had passed, leaving me wrung out and nauseous but able to sit up. Moving around a bit, I still felt that strange vacancy through my midsection, as if the middle of my torso had been drawn in chalk and then erased.

"Have you passed gas?" the nurse asked.

"Gas?"

"It sounds funny, but we can't let you go until you pass gas. Because of the laparoscopy. They expand the cavity with air. We need to know your body is getting rid of it."

She helped me stand and wobble my way to the bathroom and left me there to hopefully break wind in privacy. I waited. Nothing happened. On the other side of the heavy door, Eduardo and his parents continued their quiet conversation.

". . . now that the building is finished . . ."

". . . sooner than we . . ."

". . . competent real estate lawyers . . ."

I crept back to my bed and dozed again until I felt the nurse rubbing my arm.

"Lorena? Let's try walking, all right? Why don't you and Eduardo take a little walk down the hallway and work on releasing that air trapped inside."

Eduardo offered me his arm, and we shuffled at a snail's pace up and down the hallway, making feeble jokes.

"You break the wind beneath my wings."

70

"Till death do us fart."

Ultimately, he escorted me back to my room and then took his parents to stand uncomfortably in the hallway so I could be alone in my bed, focusing intently until I was able to expel a small *foof* of air. I was relieved, but it made me want to weep. I was supposed to be fine. I was supposed to feel better. Instead, I felt like someone who's just spent three hours trying to fart.

"I got it," I called.

The nurse came in, praised the effort accordingly, and told me the next goal was to urinate without the catheter.

"I'll bring you some supper," she said. "That might help you feel alive again."

She returned with apple juice, toast, and Jell-O. I thanked her and waited for her to leave before I pushed it aside so I could huddle into the sheets and go back to sleep. The next time I was aware of my vitals being taken, the early summer dawn had turned the windows gray.

"Will I be able to go home today?" I asked.

"We'll see. Dr. Humano needs to review your lab results."

Eduardo sat next to me and showed me a picture of the kids. They were very happy.

There was a light rap on the door before Dr. Humano opened it. (I've since noticed how everyone straightens up in their chair at the sound of that little knock, ready to be on their best behavior, as if they were in church.)

"Good morning," he said, offering Eduardo his hand. "How are you? Good to see you. Lorena, how are you feeling?"

"I'm great."

I was not great, but the words came out of my mouth before I even weighed the question. I knew the right answer, and I said it.

"Wonderful! Glad to hear it," said Dr. Humano.

He looked pleased. I could see the bald relief on Eduardo's face.

But I was not *great*. I'd been feeling a lot of things since I came to after the surgery, and *great* was not one of them.

"Actually," I said carefully, "I'm not feeling very well. I thought I'd feel better after the procedure, and I don't. I feel worse."

He listened, leaning in, nodding. "That's to be expected. You just had surgery. Get some rest. Some people need a little more time to recover. I reviewed your test results," he said, pulling up a stool. "Good news. White count, potassium level—everything's back to normal."

"Normal," I echoed. "How is that possible? I just had the surgery a few hours ago."

"Amazing, isn't it?" He smiled and opened his elegant hands in an expansive gesture. "Take out what's not working, and the body starts working again."

A surgeon's philosophy in a nutshell. Like it says in the Bible: "If thy right eye offends thee, pluck it out." I do remember wondering if this was maybe a little too good to be true, but it didn't even occur to me that my potassium level appeared normal because I'd been receiving massive doses of potassium in the IV. Maybe I was the one who could only hear what I wanted to hear in that moment, and what I wanted to hear was that I could go home.

"Am I okay to leave?" I asked.

"Good to go." He smiled.

"And . . . I'm okay to go on vacation?"

"I don't see any reason why not. The nurse will give you some instructions on how to change the dressing on your abdomen."

I pledged to follow instructions. Dr. Humano left us with a cheerful "Adios!" I got dressed and collected my things. A nurse wheeled me to the exit, and Eduardo installed me in a nest of pillows in the back seat and played soft classical music on the car stereo. I tried not to whimper, but every bump on the freeway sent a javelin of pain through my belly.

"Doing okay?" asked Tío Ricardo.

"Great," I said.

At home, Eduardo helped me up to bed and tucked me in. He looked down on me with great tenderness and such immense relief, I let myself feel relieved, too. I wanted to let it go. Have a positive attitude. Be a good patient.

He kissed me, and I said, "I'll feel better tomorrow."

I wanted to believe it truly was over. We'd look back on it and be grateful because we'd know we could get through anything together. *Sure, things are hectic now, but remember that year when Lorena wasn't doing well.* We might even laugh about some of it someday. *Till death do us fart.*

"You should go back," I told Eduardo. Blanca was there, caring for Eddie, but I didn't like the feeling of our kids so far away without me or Eduardo.

"Are you sure?"

"Yes. Absolutely. I'll come as soon as I can."

Propped up with pillows that kept me in a relatively comfortable position, I drifted through most of the day in that clammy, deadweight sleep that comes with drugs. I opened my eyes to find Tía Paty, who'd brought me a bouquet of flowers and a bowl of soup. She looked fresh and lovely in a sleeveless summer dress, which made me even more aware of my sweaty pajamas and frowsy hair. When I tried to sit up, sharp pain in my gut reminded me that my body was still processing the trapped air. My intestines were slowly returning to the task of digesting what little food and water I'd taken in. I rested my head back on the pillows and closed my eyes. Tía Paty arranged the flowers in a vase, and my stomach turned at the sickly sweet aroma.

"How are you feeling?" she asked.

"Not very well."

"Maybe it'll help to take a shower and wash your hair." She sat on the edge of the bed and smoothed a stray curl from my forehead. "You just had surgery. It'll take a few days to get back on your feet."

"I know. I just thought—"

sssssstopcomplaining

"What?" My eyes flew open. There was still a vague ringing in my ears, though it wasn't as bad as it was in the hospital. But now, just beyond it, there was the occasional shrill of a buzzy voice, like a passing mosquito. *La voz*—this little voice—stayed with me like the lingering sting of lemon on a papercut.

Tía Paty looked at me, curious and concerned. "Sweetie, what's wrong?"

"I don't know."

negative, buzzed *la voz. ssssso ungrateful*

I pressed the palm of my hand to my ear and shook my head.

"Lorena?" said Tía Paty. "What is it?"

"I don't know. I thought I heard . . . something."

sssssssheeeezzzzz so tired of you, whispered *la voz.*

"Here," said Tía Paty. "Try to drink some water."

drinkwaterdrinkwaterdrinkwater

"I don't feel well."

iiiiidontfeeeeeeelwell, *la voz* mocked.

She pressed the back of her hand to my forehead and said, "You don't seem to have a fever."

"I guess I'm just tired."

"Close your eyes," Tía Paty said. "Get some rest."

as iffffffff, buzzed *la voz.*

I was scared now, but I wasn't about to tell Tía Paty that I was hearing voices. That would sound crazy. I pretended to sleep, and she crept out quietly. Then I lay there alone, terrified, cupping and uncupping my ear with my hand, feeling like my face was on fire. It's tradition in Mexico to have a crucifix in the room above your bed, but I didn't want to sleep with all that suffering looming over me. Above the bed Eduardo and I shared, there was a spectacular painting of a shield. The artist had created a tessellation of purple, green, and blue butterfly wings radiating outward from a single small butterfly at the center. It spoke to me of rebirth and renewal, but as I lay in bed below it, I thought about birth—or rebirth—as a necessarily painful process. Perhaps I was in labor, struggling to deliver myself.

The next few days passed in a blur. Painkillers. Twisted sheets. Laborious trips from my bed to the bathroom, where I stared at my swollen belly in the mirror. The incisions were marked with crisscrossed butterfly bandages.

x marksssss the ssssssssspot

La voz was never far from my ear, buzzing her disapproval, feeding off my misery the way a mosquito would feed off a thin vein of blood. I was afraid to tell anyone because she kept reminding me of all the terrifying possibilities—psychological and spiritual—that might explain her presence. I honestly couldn't say which explanation was more frightening, demon or madness. The only thing that muffled the incessant buzz was another dose of painkillers, so I kept them ready, checking the time on my phone, counting down the minutes until I could swallow another round and crawl under the covers again. The drugs blunted my senses and sapped my energy. They made my sleep blank and dreamless. I woke feeling dizzy and ill and even more wrung out and tired than I did before I lay down, but it was worth it to shut her up for a few hours.

I understand now that auditory hallucinations—hearing voices—can be associated with imbalances in blood pressure, thyroid production, and other functions regulated by the adrenal glands. But at that moment, I truly feared I was losing my mind. Yes, it felt physical, but it also felt like encroaching dementia, the edge of madness, and my natural instinct was to do whatever I had to do to hide it.

On the third or fourth day, I made my way to the overstuffed sofa in the corner of my room, curled into a ball, and pressed my ear against the couch pillows. It was a small, agonized step toward normalcy, and I forced myself to build on it each day. My children needed me, and I would do whatever I had to do to get to them.

if they sssssssstill remember you

The following week, I went to Dr. Humano's office for the post-surgical follow-up exam. My hazy memory of that is that I felt like shit, but you wouldn't know that from Dr. Humano's notes on the occasion.

Lorena is now about a week out from a laparoscopic left adrenal-ectomy for hyperaldosteronism. Presently doing exceptionally well.

This baffles me. When I looked at these notes a year later, I wondered if he was confusing me with someone else, because this is, candidly, the least cynical conclusion I could draw in retrospect.

Hypokalemia has resolved. Blood pressure is normal. Eating well. Some anticipated retroperitoneal postoperative pain, which is not severe. Predominantly felt in the left posterior flank area as would be expected. Mild laparoscopic port incisional tenderness particularly at the 10mm transrectus port site.

I imagined him sitting at his desk, dictating these notes for a transcriptionist who would type them up and save the document to a neat file with my name on it. Done and done. In the office that day, it seemed to me that he hardly made eye contact. He brusquely skimmed the pathology report and digested the information on my behalf.

"There was apparently some nodular hyperplasia," he said. "It might indicate bilateral disorder, so we need to keep an eye on your other adrenal gland."

"Nodular hyperplasia . . . bilateral . . ." I wrote the terms down so I could Google them later. "What happens if the other adrenal gland is affected? Can you live without any adrenal glands?"

"Let's cross that bridge if we come to it."

"Am I still okay to go on this trip with my family?"

"Absolutely. No heavy lifting. Use common sense. Ask for help if you need it."

cuzzzzzzz people aren't ssssssssssick of you at all

"I'm not sure this pain medication is agreeing with me," I said. "Is there anything else you can give me?"

He wrote out a prescription and sent me on my way. I took the prescription and said nothing about the alarming voice in my head or the hot ache below my rib cage. It had been two weeks since I'd seen my children. We'd never been apart that long. I wasn't going to raise any issues that might derail my getting on that airplane in three days. I focused on the task of packing my bags.

My closet was full of flattering cocktail dresses with coordinated clutches and handbags, flowing blouses, embroidered tunics. All these things hung lifeless, a glut of intense colors and textures, and yet somehow I had nothing to wear. I couldn't bear the weight of the fabric on my shoulders. With my spinning head and heavy legs, I was too unsteady to be tottering up and down a marble staircase in heels.

ridiculousssssssssss while ssssssso many have nothing

I left the heels and cocktail dresses in the closet and filled my suitcase with sneakers, drawstring pants, and loose-fitting blouses. The pain and nausea had dulled to a deep fatigue that left me feeling weirdly detached from everything around me. I stared at the small things that usually gave me pleasure and comfort—a cup of tea, a vase of cut flowers, a freshly baked empanada—and I felt nothing. The big things I cared about, including Eduardo and my children, seemed to disappear in the distance, as if they were on a train and I were left behind on the platform. I needed to be with them again, but sorting and folding my clothes, I felt none of the excitement or joy I had expected to feel about going on this trip.

Before the surgery, I had an image in my mind of what it would be like when I joined my family. I was supposed to be fine. I was supposed to be healthy. But that scenario I imagined didn't leave time or space for healing, and there is no health without healing. I had to accept that getting "back to normal"—if there is any such thing—would take time and patience.

Three days later, I sat in the quiet kitchen waiting for my in-laws to take me to the airport and see me off. I focused my eyes on the wall where I had installed a large experimental work from a series titled *Shape Shifter* by Allora & Calzadilla. To create this piece, they glued scraps of found sandpaper on canvas in an immense grid. Each crinkled remnant holds the memory of a surface reshaped, roughness refined, or superficial color stripped away to expose the true color underneath. I can't look at it without imagining the people who did that work—manual labor typically done by immigrants—and the construction sites they transformed with their blood and muscle. When I first acquired the piece, it spoke to me about the arduous journey of people who remake the world as they go and about all the gritty moments between the freedom you dream of and the freedom you find at the end of a long, hard road. Later on, though, as I did the work of remaking my own body, it spoke to me about the destruction that must happen before a thing is built.

This magnificent work gave me courage from the moment I hung it on the wall, but when I looked at it now, *la voz* castigated me, buzzing at the back of my brain.

iffffff only you were ssssssssstrong and not obliviousss to blesssssssssings

"Quiet!" I said out loud, which did no good, but I had to try. "You are not real. This is in my mind. I can create a different reality."

get real lorena ground yoursssssssselfffffff

In the car, Tía Paty was warm and cheerful, as always, and I tried to smile and chat pleasantly. At the airport, Tío Ricardo helped me to the counter, and the gate agent sent my bags off on the conveyor belt. I hugged Tío Ricardo and went on by myself. By the time I settled into my seat, another skull-exploding Damien Hirst migraine had taken hold of my skull. I searched my bag for the new painkillers.

sure go fffffffor it . . . addictivvvvvve . . . inefffffffectivvvvvvvvve . . .

The reading light felt like a lance through my forehead, and when I reached up to shut it off, I felt the sickening pull on the incision in my abdomen. The tiny voice had a similar way of pulling at the loose threads inside me—insecurity, weakness, jealousy, self-pity, guilt—whatever it could get hold of. It was a vicious little liar, telling me that no one loved me, that I was a bad mother and a terrible person, that I was dying and going crazy.

"This is not real," I kept telling myself. "My mind is creating this."

I rubbed my cramped legs hard enough to leave bruises. I scratched my dry skin raw. I tried to read, but the words made no sense. I tried to sleep, but my mind settled into an anxious feedback loop. What if the plane had mechanical trouble? What if a storm hurled the plane down? My spirit would fly, free from this body that had so utterly betrayed me. I would fly away and know everything, and no one would know how I had failed them, how I was weak and didn't get better like I was supposed to. It terrified me how much this idea appealed to me.

I took the new painkillers from my bag and swallowed another one with a long, thirsty drink of water. *Just make it stop. Try to sleep.*

I closed my eyes and tried to envision the angel light, but in my twisted half sleep, the angels swarmed like wasps and dragged the plane down into the sea.

nine

My parents were waiting at the airport to greet me. Exhausted from the journey, I hugged and kissed them, clinging to my mother.

"Mami, I'm so glad to see you. I'm having such a hard time."

"You'll get better now. You'll be strong and healthy again in no time," she said.

Objectively, I knew I should be happy. I was here with my family, surrounded by art and nature—everything I love.

you deserve none of thisssssss

la voz reminded me over and over, like an echo in a cave.

It's hard to describe the surreal presence of this angry little buzz. It was more of a feeling than a sound. I know now that my brain was struggling to make sense of a catastrophic chemical imbalance, but at the time, I just felt fragile and attacked by a barrage of sounds and sights. Instead of love, I felt the weight of expectation when Papi said, "Let's get you home. Everyone's waiting for you."

I wanted to be with my family. At least I knew I should want that. With everyone's busy lives, it was a rare treat for us to gather like this. I knew how much it meant to Mami and Papi to have all their children and grandchildren gathered to play, eat, and be together. When we arrived, my brother and sisters waved to me from the second-floor porch. All the kiddos were tearing around the front yard, kicking a soccer ball. Everyone was happy. The accommodating host made sure everything was perfect. Eduardo hurried down the steps with the baby in his arms. Lore and Paty came running, calling, "Mommy! Mommy!"

"Watch it now," Eduardo cautioned them. "Be gentle. Mommy is still healing from her surgery."

I got down on my knees and hugged their little bodies tight against mine, kissing their cool cheeks and exclaiming how much bigger they'd gotten. Before I was ready to let go, they wriggled away, wanting to run off and play with their cousins. Eduardo helped me up and kissed me and asked, "How are you feeling?"

"Not good."

"You're here now," he said. "Everything will be all right."

Standing there with his arms around me, I could almost believe it.

Our host, Moussa, came out to greet me, offering a cold drink.

"Welcome, Lorena," he said warmly.

"Thank you."

The smell of freshly cut lemon stung my eyes.

My fingers felt thick and wooden on the cool glass.

"We're so very happy to see you. If there's anything you need, please do not hesitate to ask."

He took my suitcase, and I followed him through a great double doorway flanked by beautifully woven tapestries. I had to look away from the intricate designs so I wouldn't feel like I was falling into the thready waterfall of color and texture. There was so much history etched into the walls of the old house. I was overwhelmed at the realization. So many lives had been lived in this place. So many families had loved one another. So many souls had been born and died. I could hear music and kitchen sounds from somewhere off the wide hallway, and I took a deep breath. Black coffee, cinnamon, powdered sugar.

"Here we are. Your room, Lorena."

Moussa opened the door and followed me into the guest suite I would be sharing with my family.

thissssss art are you kidding me

"Thank you. Everything is beautiful," I said, but to be honest, the complicated decor grated on my weary soul. The aroma of fresh flowers in the hand-stenciled vases turned my stomach. Every crystal figurine felt like a needle in my eye. The four-poster bed seemed impossibly tall and inhospitable.

"Enjoy your stay," said Moussa.

He seemed disappointed. I'm sure he was used to a very different reaction, but the lovely coffered ceilings were no more comforting than all the other ceilings I'd recently been staring at.

"Please, allow me to assist you if you need help with anything at all."

sssssssssstand up straight he can sssssssee that you're crazzzzzzy

I nodded and faked a tense smile, wishing he would get out. The moment he left, softly closing the door behind him, I raced to the bathroom, violently ill. When there was nothing left in my stomach, I sat on the floor, resting my forehead on the porcelain rim of the toilet, waiting for the dry heaves to pass. I stood in the shower for a long time, trying in vain to scrape the soap scum off my skin. When I got out, all I wanted was to find a fresh T-shirt and sweats in my suitcase, climb up into the skyscraper bed, and close my eyes. The intricately beaded comforter was as heavy as lead. I managed to shape a nest for myself and find a position that protected the sensitive area around the incisions. I lay shivering, wet hair plastered to my cheek, not really sleeping, not really awake, as long afternoon shadows traveled across the floor.

It was dark when Mami knocked on the door. She seemed to have no trouble sitting up on the edge of the bed. Why was it so hard for me?

"It's dinnertime, sweetheart." My mother stroked the tangled hair away from my face. "The food here has been amazing. I don't want you to miss it."

"I'm sorry I missed the day," I said, gingerly sitting up beside her. "Jet lag, I guess."

liarliarliarliar

"Don't worry about it," she said. "Just come down and join us for dinner. Everyone will be so glad to see you."

I wrapped my shawl around my shoulders and stepped into my well-worn Uggs, but when I reached for the doorknob, I realized Mami was looking at me funny.

"Surely, you're not going to dinner like that," she said.

"It's just the family, isn't it? Do I really need to dress up?"

"Well, even if you don't want to dress up, you have to at least get dressed. Put on something nice, Lorena. It might make you feel better."

I didn't have the strength to argue. "Fine. Okay. I'll meet you down there."

"Good." She took my face between her hands and kissed my cheek. "My sweet girl. I'm glad you're here."

I'd brought a heather-gray dress I wore when I was pregnant with Eddie. It looked like a potato sack on me now, but it was loose and fairly comfortable with the shawl and Uggs. I realized I hadn't packed any makeup. Or a hairbrush. *Oh, well.*

like that would make a diffffffference

Though it was far away from our everyday lives, the place felt like home with the kids' toys scattered here and there, shoes by the door, and the smell of supper cooking. Creeping down the hall, I must have looked like a madwoman. When I came to the marble staircase, the steps warped and shifted beneath my feet. I gripped the railing and deliberately set one foot down and then the other until I reached the foyer, but there the floor was tiled with a confusing pattern of tiny squares and circles. I stepped carefully, placing my feet on the squares, because the circles seemed to spin when I looked at them, rising from the floor like flying saucers.

Yes, I thought. *This must be put right, shifted a centimeter or so. fix it fix it fix it*

I knelt down and pried at the circles with my fingernails. If I could budge it just a little, it would be perfect, and it should be perfect, because things must be perfect, and I must make everything perfect and be mathematically precise so that everything was in the correct place.

fixitfixitfixitfixitfixitfixit

fixitfixitfixitfixitfixitfixit

"Lorena? Are you all right?"

Startled, I looked up and found my sister-in-law looking down at me with the same surprise I'd seen on my mother's face a little while ago.

"What are you doing?" she asked.

she knowsssssss she can ssssssssee you're losing it

"I dropped my earring," I said. "I found it."

"Come on." She took my arm and helped me up. "Everyone's waiting for us."

I sat between Lore and one of my nephews. When I look back at pictures of our happy family dinner, I recall a beautifully set table with someone who makes me smile sitting in every chair. None of this made an impression on me at the time. I was blind to everything, including the art and the love that would have once filled my senses and brought tears to my eyes.

There was fresh baked bread and vegetables from the garden. Our hosts were knowledgeable and enthusiastic, educating us on the composition of each traditional dish. Everyone around me was laughing and enjoying the lively conversation.

"I've missed you!" My sister-in-law squeezed my hand. "How are you?"

Everyone asked me that at some point that first night. I didn't know how to answer, other than to clench my teeth and say, "Good. And you?" I mostly stayed quiet because I didn't want to talk about my heart palpitations and migraines and how the muscles in my legs knotted into cramps and charley horses every night. It's funny how the rhetorical greeting—"How are *you*?"—becomes the loaded question: "How *are* you?" I didn't want to talk about my failing body, but I hardly knew anymore how to talk about anything else. Pain and anxiety overwhelmed the vast majority of my conscious and unconscious thoughts.

We had planned a full menu of activities every day: museums, garden walks, and bicycle tours. Mami was right when she said it was everything I love, but I was unable to feel anything about any of it, and that terrified me. I was jolted awake every morning with the muscles cramping in my legs and feet. I struggled out of bed, trying to walk off the tight knots of hot pain, my heart hammering, and that tiny *la voz*, buzzing, demanding attention. The days were a test of will. The nights were endless, tossing ordeals.

One of our last evenings, the children brought everyone, young and old, together to play games, sing, and dance. It was an occasion my children will always remember. The whole lively group of family and close friends laughing and dancing, switching partners, skipping to keep up with the music. I stumbled through it, slower and less coordinated than little Eddie.

The next day I was so exhausted, I spent the day in bed while everyone else played in the pool. I heard the children dashing up and down the hallway, and Mami announced that it was time to get ready for dinner.

Get up, I scolded myself. *Just get up.*

I rolled onto my side and forced myself to sit up and drag the shawl across my shoulders. I immediately wanted to lie down again, but I knew people were expecting me.

I didn't bother to brush my teeth or change my clothes. I opened the door and found Mami in the hallway, meticulously beautiful in a crisply ironed fuchsia blouse. Her hair cascaded to her shoulders. Her lips were painted.

tsssk tssk, *la voz* chided, *clearly she is sssssso disappointed in you*

"Mami, can't I just have dinner in my pajamas? Please. I don't feel well."

Her pink lips tightened to a frown, and she sighed a deeply disheartened sigh.

My mother's unshakable love for me is one of the few things I have always been sure of. There has not been a single moment of my life in which I doubted her complete devotion and utterly dependable ability to care for and comfort me. More than anything I wanted to tell her what was happening to me, but I couldn't bear to worry and disappoint her. My "recent surgery" excuse wasn't cutting it anymore. People who loved me needed me to be myself again. They didn't have to say it out loud. I knew what they were thinking. "Get over it, Lorena. You're fine. The doctor said so."

As Mami disappeared down the hallway, I went back to my room and wedged myself into a pair of linen pants with a striped blouse. I put on pearl earrings and a gold necklace and forced a comb through my wild hair. I started down the marble stairs before I remembered that I must avoid the staircase with the spinning tiles at the bottom. Suddenly, I was standing there in the middle of that weirdly gyrating floor. Moussa was standing in the doorway. He watched me walk in circles for a moment before he cleared his throat and said, "Lorena? May I help you?"

"These tiles are wrong," I said. "I need to change these tiles."

"Tiles?"

"The floor. The circles. Look at them! Don't you see? If you just rearrange—they're not right. We have to make them right."

"Lorena?" My sister-in-law came to the hallway and set her hand on my elbow. "What's wrong?"

Moussa's voice was clipped and cold. "She wants me to move the floor."

ice burn who doesssss he think he issssssss

"What?" She laughed, assuming he must have misunderstood me. "Come on. Let's go to dinner."

Clutching her arm, I went to the dining room and sat through the boisterous family meal hardly making eye contact with anyone else at the table. I couldn't bear to look at Mami, fearing I'd see the disappointment in her eyes. I couldn't face Moussa, certain he must be snickering about the weird lady who demanded he move the floor. My sisters tried to engage me in conversation. Paty danced over to show me her crown of flowers from the garden. Lore wanted to say something for me in Mandarin. I responded with all the sparkling personality of a zombie.

Eventually, the clanking of silverware and clatter of plates was too much. I had to leave. As I hurried to my room, the very walls seemed to be crashing down around me. I felt as if the house itself were trying to swallow me up, consume me, crush me. I dashed across the tiles, afraid that if I looked at them one more time, I would have to take a hammer to them.

fixitfixitfixitfixitfixitfixitfixit

I tried to outrun her, but *la voz* followed me to my room and slithered under the covers. Even in the dark under the duvet, I felt spikes of light in my eyes. The migraine screamed through my head like a jet plane landing. I was going to throw up. The sheets tangled around my legs as I struggled free and dashed to the bathroom where I vomited until I was wrung hollow.

A little while later, I found myself standing in front of the mirror, staring at the running water. I couldn't remember what I was supposed to do next. I heard the bedroom door open and close softly. Eduardo reached past me and shut off the water.

"Lorena, what's wrong?"

"I don't know. *Mi amor*, I don't know. I had the surgery. I did everything exactly as I was told to do it."

"You're recovering. It takes time."

"No. No. They said I was supposed to be okay, and I'm not okay. I'm *worse*. I don't know what's happening. Something is horribly wrong with me."

don't sssssay it keep it a sssssecret

he won't love you

This I knew was a lie. With his arms around me, I was able to say it out loud. "*Mi amor*, I'm losing my mind. I'm going crazy."

The truth tumbled out with a flood of tears. As I described what had been happening to me since the day I left the hospital, I could see the tears welling in Eduardo's eyes as well. In all our years together, I could count on one hand the number of times I'd seen him cry, and he cried now. Grief-stricken and afraid, we wept together for what seemed like a long time, standing in the bathroom for a while and then huddled together on the bed.

"Do you think it's depression?" he asked.

"I can't believe this is all in my head. It feels real. It feels physical."

I wasn't sure it made any difference, putting a label on this looming darkness that had taken over my life. The words no longer mattered. I no longer trusted my own perception of reality.

"Whatever it is," said Eduardo, "we'll fight it together. You'll be okay."

no you won't, la voz whispered. *you will never be okay again*

"You'll be okay," everyone kept telling me, and I kept biting back the question, *What if I'm not?* It was unthinkable. I couldn't bear to fail my family. More than anything I wanted to be a strong, healthy mother for my children. I wanted to be the dependable partner Eduardo believed in—the fully alive woman with whom he had fallen in love. The way he looked at me now broke my heart because I knew I was breaking his. If there was anything I could have done to calm his fears and take those tears from his eyes, I would have done it.

But the hard truth is, you can't force yourself to be *okay* for someone else just because they need or want you to be okay. You can pretend for a while—wax-drip that "positive attitude" over your pain—but it's not sustainable. There's nothing healthy or courageous about faking a smile and putting on some facade of normalcy. Even the mask of medication is bound to crack as the body builds tolerance, refusing to be ignored.

Troubles put a microscope on all our relationships. Whatever was there to start with will be magnified. A strong foundation becomes invincible. The fissures in a cracked foundation will widen. The foundational relationships in my life were good, I'm glad to say, but only when I had the courage to share what was really happening to me. It wounded my pride to be the one in need, and it wounded his pride that he couldn't fix this for me. Ultimately, we would have to learn to need each other, and he would have to respect my ability to fix things for myself.

Sometimes it's hard for people who love us to accept that we are simply *not okay*. They may think they're helping or encouraging—*Get up! Take a shower! Put on something nice and you'll feel better!*—because they want more than anything for you to be the strong person they've always believed you to be. But when I tried to be that person, I found myself sitting on the shower floor, watching the water swirl and circle the dark holes in the drain.

I know that if I had ever asked my mother point-blank— "Mami, do you want to know the truth about me or do you want me to pretend?"—she would never want me to lie to her, and she would have been strong enough to accept the truth, even though the truth was painful for both of us. Given the opportunity, she would have immediately embraced and supported me, but having seen her world so recently shattered by Roby's cancer diagnosis, I couldn't bring myself to pile a fresh disaster on top of her. I was haunted by the sound of that disconsolate wail.

It would have been lovely to have my family on my side in those weeks following the surgery, but they never really had a chance to respond to what was actually happening. They didn't have all the information. I sent them off, proudly declaring I would handle this on my own, and then when it all went terribly wrong, I was afraid to confide in them. I was ashamed of my craziness, my weakness, my failure to live up to everyone's expectations.

Lore, Paty, and Eddie have happy memories of this trip. They remember happy family meals, bike rides, games. All credit for that goes to my family, along with kindhearted Moussa, who took care of us all and even took a turn on the swing when the children begged him to.

Flying home, I felt hopeless and bereft.

I didn't know if I would ever be myself again. Even if I was able to get past all this, what would be left of me when I got to the other side? I thought I'd failed my family, failed myself, even failed my wonderful surgeon by not getting better.

It never even occurred to me that the surgeon had, in fact, failed me.

ten

Eduardo was still commuting to Monterrey for work, so Blanca and I went to South Padre with my mother and sisters and all the children, planning to stay until it was time for the kiddos to go back to school at the end of August. Eduardo joined us on the weekends, and I was always relieved to see him. He was the only one who had even a vague idea about the pain and misery that had all but overwhelmed me.

The condo was filled with unopened boxes, things I'd ordered or shipped from home the year before when I still had energy and ideas. Filled with happy anticipation, I'd sketched and shopped and planned, looking forward to preparing the place for a joyful summer. But now the July heat beat down, thick and humid. The art I had carefully curated seemed flat and uninspired. The pillows were the wrong shape. The furniture didn't fit, no matter how I shifted it. Even if I'd had the energy to execute the design I'd originally envisioned, I no longer felt any passion for that or anything else.

Still, it was a relief to be in a place that felt like home. I could wear my pajamas all day if I felt like it. I could lie down in the shade and listen to my children play. The ambient sound of the sea was comforting and consistent. The voice in my head receded into the background for the most part. I felt a surge of hope. Maybe I was getting better. I made myself open the boxes, put towels in the linen closet and bedding on the beds. Unpacking the embroidered tea towels and sofa pillows, I felt no joy, but the mechanics kept me going, and that was something.

I searched through the cardboard and bubble wrap until I found three quartz crystals I'd sent to myself. The weight of them in my arms was as comforting as the sound of the sea. Here was something ancient, unchangeable, and incorruptible that anchored me to that person I was before it all began. I set them on the kitchen island and went to lie down on the sofa. The small effort of unboxing these few items left me wiped out. It was like moving mountains.

One of the random items I'd unpacked was a photo album my mother had given me. It was filled with family pictures from our traditional Christmas celebration the year before Eddie was born. In those pictures, I was laughing, playing with my children, and reveling in all the holiday cheer. The tree was full of fairy lights. Lore and Paty wore sweet little dresses with snowflakes and lace. I looked slender and fit in a tailored velvet blouse and rich red lipstick. Sarcastic little *la voz* had a good time taunting me about that.

"Good morning, Lorena!"

I heard the kitchen door open and then the *click clock* of Mami's sandals on the tile floor. I tried to ignore the way my heart skipped and reeled.

"Goodness," she said, whisking the curtains aside. "Why is it so dark in here on a beautiful day like today?"

I shielded my eyes from the light. "Mami, please don't."

"Are the kids still asleep? I was hoping to have breakfast with them before they run outside. Once they get out on the beach with their cousins, I won't have another minute to keep them all to myself." She sat on the arm of the sofa and touched my forehead with the back of her hand. "How are you feeling today?"

"Heavy," I said.

Not understanding that I meant heavy like lead, she said, "You're beautiful as you are, but maybe you'll feel better if you lose a few pounds. Why don't we start walking together?"

"It's not that kind of heaviness. It's like there's gravity inside me, pulling me down. My face, my feet, my arms—everything. I feel like I might burst open and spill. Every little noise makes me feel like I'm going to have a heart attack."

"Do you feel like there's a fat man sitting on your chest?" she asked. "Like something very heavy is crushing you?"

"Sometimes."

"Maybe it's an anxiety attack."

"Maybe."

"Or it could be hormones—baby blues staying too long or the change coming too early." She stopped herself when she saw the tears in my eyes. She took me into her arms the way she would take one of the little kids. Looking back on it, I see how hard she was trying, wanting to help me, but at the time, that little voice kept hissing at me.

why mussssst you be sssssssssssuch a burden

"Mami, I don't want to be this way. It's really scaring me."

"I know it's been hard," she said, "but you're going to get through this."

"I will. I promise. I just wish it would be soon."

"It will be. The surgery is done—"

"The surgery made it *worse*. I don't know how, but it did."

"The doctor says all your tests are normal. They know what they're doing. Think how quickly Roby was able to be on her feet again."

It was her loving way of saying, "Suck it up, buttercup!"—which is exactly what I was saying to myself. I stood in front of the mirror every night, looking myself directly in the eye, telling myself,

"Lorena. You are loved. You are lovable. You are strong. Snap out of it! You are creating this reality. Make this disappear."

I knew what I felt like when I was my better self, and I was determined to will that self back into being. Who has surgery and gets *worse*? I didn't see how that was possible.

Renu reminded me that it's all connected—body, mind, and spirit—though surgeons and doctors never seem to treat the whole person. She recommended a doctor who specialized in integrative medicine, so I tried that. I learned about Marma therapy, acupressure, and moxibustion, which incorporates smoldering herbs. I'd given up on the idea of an all-encompassing diagnosis. I no longer believed in a "cure" for whatever was wrong with me. My objective now was to manage my symptoms, striving for some kind of holding pattern where the pain and despair were less overwhelming.

Renu gave me hormone cream and herbal supplements, and I did feel a small improvement. Or maybe I was imagining that *la voz* seemed to sleep most of the time, only coming out at her most vicious when I was tired or had a migraine. I prayed, meditated, and consciously practiced gratitude and patience, spending hours beneath a particular tree, a massive old oak with a gnarled trunk and twisted limbs. I sat on the mossy exposed roots that lay on top of the ground and imagined the extensive invisible root system down below. *This is how life is*, I reminded myself. *What you see is only a fraction of what you get. There is always so much more than you know.*

Cicadas sang in the oppressive Texas heat. I managed my days with a strict energy budget. I knew exactly how much I could do before my body rebelled, and it wasn't much, but I tried to get the most I could from it. I strategized each move from bed to sofa and back to bed, and I tried to take pleasure in small accomplishments and pleasures, inching forward with the renovation of the condo—a project I'd planned with such happy anticipation. More than ever before, I was aware of how important it was to preserve the flow of peaceful energy around me. I was hyperaware of anything out of place, hypersensitive to clashing patterns and conflicting colors. For the first time in my life, I was afraid of stimulation, rather than craving it. I'd always been an adventurous artist, ready to experiment. Now I had to conserve my capacity for frustration, which is sad, because a willingness to screw up and start over is vital to any artist—and any human being.

In the hallway between Eddie's nursery and the bedroom shared by Lore and Paty, I began work on an installation featuring hammered brass eggshells, similar to the whimsical ant installation on the stairway wall in our living room in Austin. I marked out the arrangement of the eggshells, labeling the location for each one with a carpenter's pencil, and used a power drill to bolt the first two or three to the wall. The noise and vibration were more than I could stand. Leaving the pieces scattered on the floor, I went out to the beach and waved to Lore and Paty, who played in the water while Eddie drove a toy dump truck through the sand.

Blanca had gone to visit her family, so Mari, my nanny, was watching them the same way she watched over me when I was a little girl. The sand was hot, the tide pools as warm as bathwater. The Gulf of Mexico stretched to the horizon under an intensely blue sky. Eduardo was due to fly in later that evening, looking forward to a quiet family weekend.

"Mommy," Paty called, "watch me do a handstand!"

She dived into the water, and a moment later her feet stuck straight up above the gentle waves. Then her feet disappeared, and her head popped up again.

I applauded. "Amazing! Are you getting hungry?"

"Yes!"

This is a trick question. My crew is always hungry at the beach. They play so hard, it's a wonder they can take in as many calories

97

as they burn off each day. With Lore in the lead, the three of them raced for the door.

"I should go into Brownsville," I said to Mari. "Why don't you come with me? We could take the kids to lunch and run a few errands before Eduardo gets home. It would really help me if you'd come with us."

"Of course." She got up and brushed sand from her skirt.

Brownsville, the nearest town of any real size, was about forty-five minutes from the beach, so by the time we got there, the kids were starving and restless. I pulled into a Red Lobster, the first place I saw where I could get them something other than fast food. We crossed the searing-hot parking lot to the door, where I was hit with a blast of cold air from the AC. I felt the temperature shift like a blow to the back of my head. The kids scrambled into a booth, and I focused on their faces, trying to avoid the visual clang of the bright red upholstery.

When the waitress came, I ordered food for the kids and said, "Just water for me, please. No ice." As they gobbled their lunch, I sat with the glass between my hands, breathing, mindful, happy to be with them. When it was time to go, we pushed through the door into the heat of a Texas August afternoon. It felt like a coal furnace. Lore and Paty scrambled into the back seat, yelping at the burning-hot buckles on their seat belts. I lifted Eddie into his toddler seat. He squirmed and howled. The sound went through my head like a thunderbolt.

"Mari," I said. And then my face was close to the gritty pavement, the tarry smell of asphalt close to my nose. I tried to get up. Couldn't. I felt the sting of cement on my knees. When I looked down at my hand, it disintegrated into a swirl of gray particles. I heard Mari's voice. She called my name and spoke to me in Spanish. I could feel her arms, and then I felt her dragging on my purse, searching for my phone.

My body was hot and then cold. My head was heavy and then light.

I wanted to tell Mari to take care of my children. I wanted to tell my children that I loved them. No words. No air. Only the mournful wail of sirens in the distance.

eleven

The hospital record states time of arrival was 14:58, just a few minutes before three in the afternoon: *Thirty-three-year-old Hispanic Female presents to ER with complaints of dizziness. 14:58: Patient presents with feeling faint. Onset: Symptoms / episode began / occurred two weeks ago. Context: Occurred outdoors, occurred while the patient was walking, just prior to the episode the patient experienced abdominal pain, light-headedness, difficulty breathing. Symptoms began when she was vacationing. Modifying factors: symptoms are alleviated by nothing, symptoms are aggravated by movement of head, standing up, changing position. Associated signs and symptoms: pertinent positives: abdominal pain. Pertinent negatives: confusion, headache, numbness, vomiting.*

I find it odd that the surgery isn't mentioned. Apparently, I was in no shape to supply the correct information. I was vaguely aware of the lights in the ER, the rolling motion of the gurney, and then a spray of flowers in a vase near the spot in the hallway where they parked me. I could smell the rose petals moldering, past their prime. The smell of death and decay. I lay waiting, balanced on the edge of consciousness. I woke to find Mami and Roby standing over me, their faces full of worry and frustration.

"My kids," I said. "Where are they?"

"With Tía Paty," said Mami. "Don't worry." (Tía Paty and Tío Ricardo had a condo in South Padre, too.)

"They're fine," said Roby. "Just a little scared. I told them Mommy will be okay."

A nurse came and took me for a CT scan.

"I don't like all this radiation," Mami said as they wheeled me away. "She's been through so much already."

The nurse brought me back after the scan, and we sat together—Mami, Roby, and me—weighed down by the feeling that we'd all been here before. It was not an upscale place, as ERs go. The pale curtains were faded and thin. There were greasy fingerprints on the metal table. A fluorescent bulb flickered and hummed over our heads, warning that it was due to burn out. Right after Mami excused herself and went to take a phone call, the doctor arrived.

It's funny, I now have no memory of his name or face. I only remember that he was a small, dapper Indian gentleman. And I remember what he told me: "We found a 1.4-centimeter tumor on your right adrenal gland."

"No. That can't be right." I sat up, unsteady, trying to make sense of it.

"Here." He turned the computer screen toward me and pointed with the tip of his pen to a distinct, dark knot on the grainy image. "You can see it right there. I see you had the left gland surgically removed. When was that?"

"About four weeks ago."

"Adrenal tumors are rarely malignant, but I can tell from your blood work—low potassium, etcetera—it's definitely active. You need to get it removed as soon as possible."

Roby and I exchanged an agonized glance. This was the same thing Dr. Blevins had told me before. *Exactly* the same. Like a recurring nightmare.

"Your endocrinologist in Austin," he said. "That would be . . ."

"Dr. Blevins."

"Blevins." He nodded and wrote that down. "I'll give him a call and forward these scans so you can follow up with him."

"But what about—" I started, but he was already on his way out.

"Follow up with Dr. Blevins," he said. "I'm sorry. I need to get to the next patient."

Roby and I stood there, stunned by the whole thing—the bombshell, the abrupt departure, the unimaginable coincidence of the exact same diagnosis.

"Lorena, are you okay?" She nudged me back to my chair. "You should sit."

"I've been trying to tell people—no one would believe me—and then he tells me, but then he leaves. No one is willing to *help* me."

Roby grasped my hand. "I'm here, Lorena. I want to help."

"What's wrong?" Mami stepped inside the curtained cubicle. "Was that the doctor leaving just now? What did he say?"

I told her, and she shook her head in disbelief.

"Dr. Humano said the pathology report indicated a bilateral condition," I said, "but I didn't think it could be so soon."

I covered my face with my hands, trying to imagine how I would tell Eduardo. My mother set a protective arm around me, shifting into crisis management mode.

"Let's go back to the condos," she said. "Eduardo will be there this evening. We'll pack our things and go home to Austin tomorrow. You'll see Dr. Humano, and he'll fix this."

So that was the plan. I had nothing else to suggest. On the long ride back to South Padre, I huddled in the back seat, mourning this new development, despairing. This was never going to get better.

My children would grow up without a functional mother. Lore's and Paty's childhood memories would be split into two eras: before Mommy got sick and after Mommy got sick. Eddie would have no memories at all in which I was my real self.

We arrived at Tía Paty's high-rise building, and she came out to meet us. She put her arms around me and reassured me that the kids had been happily playing all afternoon. I was about to follow her inside when I felt my cell phone buzz.

"It's Dr. Blevins," I said. "I need to take it."

"Of course. Come up when you're ready."

I nodded and took the call. "Hi, Dr. Blevins. Sorry to bother you again."

"It's no bother, Lorena. Not at all," he said, but he sounded a little uptight.

"The thing is, I fainted, and they took a CT scan at the ER—"

"Yes." He cleared his throat. "Lorena, I'm here with Dr. Humano."

"Oh. He's there?"

"Dr. Humano needs to tell you something."

There was a brief shuffle on the other end of the line, and then Dr. Humano said, "Hi, Lorena. This is Dr. Humano."

I felt relief when I heard his voice. Here was someone who leaned in and listened to me, someone who made decisions and took incisive action. And while Dr. Blevins sounded oddly uptight, Dr. Humano's tone was relaxed and sociable.

"Hey, how are you feeling?" he said.

"Not great, to be honest. I've had a very hard time adjusting since—"

"Yes. Well. After surgery, you know, it takes time. The body needs time to recover."

"Yes. I know," I said. Me. Aka "the body." Standing there on the sidewalk, I shaded my eyes from the sun and waited for him to say something else.

"So. How was your trip?" he said.

"Very nice," I answered mechanically. "Thank you for asking."

"Good. Very good." He sounded totally chill making this small talk. As if this was all par for the course. As if I hadn't just left the ER with a fresh dose of rotten news. "So . . . yes. Lorena, we saw the results from your scan today—Dr. Blevins and I. The Brownsville facility had all the details sent over."

"I didn't think it could happen so soon. The bilateral—"

"No," he cut in. "It's not that. Lorena, this is—I don't know quite how to tell you this." He took a deep breath. "I took out the wrong side."

My whole world distilled to a tight ball of intense heat and light. I stood at the center of it, trying to parse the words I was hearing, thinking he could not possibly be saying what I thought he was saying.

I said, "I don't understand."

"I took the wrong adrenal gland."

"But what about . . . *what?*" I tried to swallow. My throat felt sandy and raw. "What are you saying?"

"I don't know how it happened. We should have taken the right. We took the left. If you would like to come to my office tomorrow—if you have any questions—we could talk."

I didn't know how to respond. *If* I had *questions?*

"So that is the situation. Please make an appointment to see me as soon as possible. And know that I love you."

I flinched from the sound of clumsy disconnect. I don't remember if either one of us actually said "goodbye." I sank down to sit on the sidewalk. Someone with normal adrenal glands would have received an electrifying jolt of energy then. Adrenaline is one of the body's great coping mechanisms, specifically engineered for a moment like this. I would have been grateful for it. Instead, I recognized the shrill ringing in my ears, a crushing fullness in my head that I now knew was my unregulated blood pressure, wildly out of control. Feeling like I might pass out, I lay down with my cheek to the warm pavement and stayed there for a little while, looking on a world turned sideways. I don't know if anyone saw me there like that. If they did, I didn't care.

Eventually, I felt stable enough to get up and stumble to my car. I dug my keys from my purse and started the engine so I could turn on the AC, and then I dug for my phone, cool air blowing on my flushed red face and neck.

Tía Paty answered immediately. "Lorena, is everything all right?"

"I don't know. I need to go home. Can you keep the kids? Eduardo will be here tonight. He'll come and get them in the morning."

There was a pause while she waited for me to volunteer additional information, and when I didn't, she said, "We're here. Whatever you need."

"Thank you."

I probably shouldn't have been driving, but it wasn't far. All I could think about at the moment was getting home, and when I got home, I sat in the twilight and cried. A velvet curtain of grief descended on me. There's no shortcut through the stages of grief—denial, anger, depression, bargaining, and acceptance—and it seemed at first that all these reactions were on the spin cycle. *La voz* snapped and shrieked in a feedback loop.

sssssssso messssssed up sssssssso messssssed up sssssssso messssssed up

For the first time, the tiny voice was powerless. It couldn't terrify me anymore. I was not crazy. I was not weak. I was right—*I was right!*—when I tried to tell people that I had gotten worse after the surgery. Never again would other people—or even a voice inside my own head—make me doubt myself or deny what I was feeling. A nine is a freaking *nine*, and I would never again be shamed into pretending it was less than that. From now on, I would be the world's foremost authority on *Lorena's body*. I would be the CEO of *Lorena*, and anyone I employed to consult on or care for my body would have to earn my trust.

The balcony doors were open, and a spectacular late-summer twilight filled the windows that faced the Gulf. I sat still, listening to the rhythm of the outgoing tide, watching the colors deepen from bright blue to hazy purple and finally to an inky black night dotted with stars and yard lights. The shrill ringing in my ears ebbed with the twilight, and I felt strangely calm by the time I heard Eduardo's key in the door.

"Anyone home?" He gave a bright whistle that usually brought the kids running. He always drops his briefcase and coat, like the unsaddling of a horse, so his arms are wide open by the time they get to him.

"I'm here," I said.

"What's up? Why is it so dark?"

"I need you to listen," I said. "And I need you to not get angry and react in a visceral, primitive way."

"What's happening?" He flipped a light switch, and when he saw me sitting there—shawl clutched tight around my shoulders, eyes red from weeping—I felt his guard go up. "Just tell me."

I told him. I laid out the bones of the information for him as plainly and dispassionately as I could. "Dr. Humano made a mistake. He took my healthy adrenal gland. The one with the tumor is still inside me."

Eduardo stared for a moment, struggling to assimilate the information the same way I had, and then he made a sound like someone had punched him in the neck.

"That's not—how could—*what?* Tell me exactly what he said. His exact words."

"He said he doesn't know how it happened and that—I don't remember exactly—that I should come to his office. And that he loves me."

Repeating it all made it even more incomprehensible. *Know that I love you?* What did that even mean? In what universe is that an appropriate substitute for *I'm sorry*?

Eduardo roared, beyond livid, beyond grief-stricken. He paced like a wounded lion in a cage. "We will sue him. I swear that—"

"Stop." I pushed my fingertips against my temples. "*Mi amor*, I need you to stop. I need to figure out the next step."

"The next step is that we sue him and take his medical license."

"First, I have to figure out how to *survive* this! I'm not thinking about a lawsuit or anything else until I figure out how I can *live* and take care of our kids and be healthy again—or at least as healthy as I can be. Instead of raging around telling me what you're going to do, I need you to *listen*. I need you to stay calm and *help me*."

He nodded, pushing a clenched fist against his mouth, physically collecting himself. I'd never seen anyone so angry. When he came and sat next to me, we were both trembling.

"Do your parents know?" he asked quietly.

I shook my head. "Only you and me. I need to get the information before I try to talk to anyone about it."

I went to the kitchen for my iPad. Eduardo used his laptop. Before the surgery, my research was all about living with one adrenal gland. Now we tried to find what we could about living with none.

Over the course of the evening, we made the necessary calls. In my family, when something is happening, everyone has to be informed. Everyone gets to weigh in with their response, and in this case, the response was exactly what you would expect. Outrage. Long, loud, profanity-filled outrage. If there's ever a moment in which I doubt my family's love for me, I'll still have the echo of all that swearing in my ears to remind me.

I'd never seen or heard Eduardo's father raise his voice about anything. He was unflappable, a properly cordial gentleman without fail, but just like his son, Tío Ricardo sucked in a deep, gut-punched breath and let loose a stream of angry words and invectives. Universally furious, tearful with wrath on my behalf, my family—the most loving, generous, kindhearted people I know—immediately went to the same place Eduardo did: *We need to sue him!*

I suppose this is evolution, in a way. We feel the same emotion our protohuman ancestors did, the same impulse to lash out, but now instead of clubs, we carry cell phones. The fight-or-flight instinct is as strong as it ever was, but the resources have changed. For me, flight was not an option and fight stole from my precious store of available energy. All that rage swirling around me was the opposite of what I needed, but I realized that I had to step back and let the people who love me process this in their own way. At the core of Eduardo's anger was his devotion to me. My mother's wrath was the snarl of a mama bear protecting her cub. Eventually, I would learn to hear it that way.

It was well after midnight when Eduardo and I lay down to sleep, and I was up at three in the morning. The potassium they gave me in the ER was taking effect, but the muscles in my calves and feet felt perilously close to clamping down in cramps and charley horses. Trying to walk it off, I crept barefoot to the kitchen. I poured breakfast cereal into a bowl and sat stirring the flakes around in the milk, thinking about Dr. Humano, replaying the conversation over and over in my head. I could see him standing there in Dr. Blevins's office, Adam's apple bobbing as he swallowed his nerves and blurted out the truth. And then what? Did he go home? Did he go out to dinner? He was home by now, no doubt, sleeping soundly, and in the morning, he would go to the hospital and operate on someone else. Someone who trusted him. Someone who was comforted by his lanky, graceless stride and his meticulously elegant hands.

My cereal had gone soggy. I poured it into the garbage disposal, picked up my cell phone, and texted Dr. Blevins.

Hola, Doctor. I'm not sure what to do next. Please, can you help me?

I slept for a few uneasy hours and woke to find his answer:

Yes, Lorena, I am going to do all I can to help. I need you to come back to Austin. We can reevaluate here.

I didn't reach out to Dr. Humano. I was more than a little stunned that he never reached out to me. Not that evening, not the next day, or the following week, or month, or year. No apology. No explanation. No referrals. No *just checking to see if you're okay.*

In the weeks and months that followed that shattering phone call, as I gathered and pored over my medical records, I would come to understand what Dr. Humano could not explain to me that day. When Dr. Blevins had my abdomen scanned, the radiologist noted the tumor on the *right* adrenal gland. Throughout their report, they referred to the tumor on the *right* adrenal gland, and the scans clearly showed the tumor on the *right* adrenal gland. But in one line at the very end of the report, there was a typo. It said, *Conclusion: Remove left adrenal gland.*

I can't say with certainty that Dr. Humano never looked at the scans or read the full report, but it appears to me that instead of reading the report and looking at the scans, he jumped to that little one-line conclusion, which happened to be the one line that contained the wrong information. *TLDR*, as they say. *Too long, didn't read.* Isn't that why God created conclusions? So that people who are terribly busy and important won't be bothered with the tedious chore of getting correct information? How could he have failed to view the full report, I wondered, and why had *I* never seen it myself? I certainly would have read it carefully, if I'd known it existed. Was it standard procedure to assume that I was better off without this information or simply incapable of digesting it?

I don't know the phase of the moon or what the traffic was like the day of my surgery. I don't know if Dr. Humano kissed his wife or tossed a ball for his dog on his way out the door. I don't know what was playing in his earbuds or playing through his mind that might have distracted him. I'm certain there was no malice, no ill will or desire to hurt me. I would think that when Dr. Blevins broke the news to him, Dr. Humano probably felt a bit of the surrealistic horror I felt when he broke the news to me, but—unlike me—he could walk away whole and move on from his mistake. I did not walk away whole. Part of me was lost. Not just part of my body, part of my *self*. Because, as Renu had reminded me, the body, mind, and spirit could not be separated.

"When the spirit doesn't get it," she said, "it goes to emotion, and when emotion doesn't get it, it goes to the body."

Now I saw wholeness as a process of reverse engineering that perfect design. I would have to start with my body and work my way up.

twelve

There are moments that change everything, and there are moments that change our *perception* of everything. I suddenly understood this important difference. The moment Dr. Humano took my healthy adrenal gland and left the tumor, I descended into a nightmare in which the world made sense and I was crazy—as if I were trying to run up the down escalator. The moment I learned the truth, everything shifted into reverse. I could see now that, in fact, the situation was crazy and all my physical and emotional reactions to it had made perfect sense. This is the essence of enlightenment—understanding that perception is power—so even though I felt body-slammed by this bad news, I woke up the next morning keenly aware that the truth had set me free. Instead of groping around in the dark, I could pick myself up and move in a healing direction.

No one enjoys receiving bad news, but ignorance is an incubator in which bad things become worse. Information is healthy, even when it feels like a body slam. (Apply as needed to parenting, politics, and life in general.)

For weeks, I'd been scolding myself in the mirror: "You are creating this reality, Lorena. You have the power to change it." Now I knew. This harsh reality had been created for me by Dr. Humano, and I had the power to change only one thing: myself. Now, armed with this brutally correct information, I could start over, and this time I would be in charge. I would never again second-guess my sanity or back-burner my concerns, operating on the assumption that a doctor knows what's best for me. I value wise advice from my parents and husband, and it makes good sense to consult experts, but going forward, I would ask questions, gather information, listen to differing opinions, and then make my own decision.

Eduardo and I spent a quiet morning, each of us deep in thought and up to our noses in research. Before breakfast, my parents were on my doorstep, ready for action, and we all gathered at the kitchen island with our laptops open.

"I was up all night reading," Mami said. "There's a study at Harvard about adrenal tissue regeneration. We need to find out more about that. And they're experimenting with transplants, so hopefully in the future, I can give you one of my adrenal glands."

This is how Mami thinks of her children. There's no part of herself she would hold back. She wouldn't hesitate. But the transplant was a hypothetical at the time.

"It's possible to survive without adrenal glands," I said. "It's not ideal, but according to what I've read, with chemical substitutes and constant blood work, they can make it better than it has been."

Eduardo and my father were already discussing the assembly of a legal team.

"We have to start thinking about the next steps," said Eduardo. "Medical records, expert testimony—there's a lot involved."

My father nodded. "I'll make some calls today."

My brother arrived, bringing tacos for breakfast, and the four of them engaged in a lively discussion of how this was going to go down. I listened without chiming in. It seemed to be a foregone conclusion that the natural response to this situation was to sue this doctor, but I was in survival mode.

"I can't think about all that right now," I said when I could get a word in. "I'm not making any decisions until I have a plan in place for this next surgery and whatever comes after that, then I'll think about whether or not I want to sue him."

"I support you if you sue him," my brother said. "Why would you not? He's in business. You were his client. He screwed up. There are consequences. He should get what he deserves."

"Does anyone ever get what they deserve?" I wondered. "Good or bad?"

"This is no time to be philosophical. This is the time for action," said Mami.

On this we could agree. I said, "I'll think about it, I promise, but my first priority is finding a way forward with another surgeon."

It was hard for me to switch gears and suddenly start thinking of Dr. Humano as my enemy. I was angry, obviously, but what is justice in a matter like this one? I honestly didn't know. If justice is balance, how could that be achieved? I had been robbed of my adrenal gland. How do you attach a dollar value to that? If an adrenal gland could be purchased at any price, I'd have one right now. Believe me, I tried. I was a beggar with a bagful of money. And yes, money can solve a multitude of problems. But not this one.

The most precious things in my life—energy, strength, sanity, time—these things are not for sale. Every ounce of my stamina was dear to me now. How would it benefit my family if I invested what little I had in fighting for something as esoteric as *justice*? It's easy to believe in grand ideals in theory, but when you're a young mama with little children, there are shoes to be tied, school papers to be crowed over, tangled hair to be combed, diapers to be changed—a 24-7 cascade of small, tender moments. My children had to be my first priority now. What little fight was left in me now was reserved for this tumor. My first order of business was finding the right person to help me get rid of it.

Back to Dr. Blevins's office. I sat in the familiar chair beneath the melancholic gaze of the grass-munching longhorn. Our first priority was to bring some semblance of control to the rampant symptoms I'd been living with. He prescribed a buffet of drugs and hormones, including heart medication to regulate my racing pulse. Almost immediately, *la voz* faded, the migraines ebbed, and my potassium-starved muscles stopped seizing. After all those weeks of suffering, this was sweet relief. I tried not to think about how needless all that suffering turned out to be.

I spent hours researching how the pharmaceuticals reacted with the Ayurvedic remedies that seemed to be helping. This wasn't a long-term solution, only a plateau where I could stop for a few weeks and regain some equilibrium. I hated the stifling effect of all these drugs. I felt sluggish and emotionally numb, and my limbs swelled with water weight. But with blood pressure, potassium, and other factors in a holding pattern, I could safely pause to consider my options.

My first impulse was to want the second surgery immediately, but I'd rushed in last time, insisting that I couldn't wait, accepting the first recommendation offered. This time, I would take it slow, gather more information, and let a cooler head prevail. I discussed my options with Eduardo, the one person whose daily life would be directly impacted by the results of my decisions.

"We have to move ahead carefully," he said. "We can't shoot and miss again."

I read everything I could get my hands on, consulted with medical experts and with people I trusted for frank, broad-minded opinions.

When I told Renu what had happened, she was horrified, but she didn't waste time on pity or panic. She dived into research on the possibility of a partial adrenalectomy—a possibility that had never been considered when the tumor was originally diagnosed. When I had asked Dr. Humano if it was possible, he had brushed the idea aside, citing the awkward position and rich blood supply to the adrenal gland. After all, he had reassured me, I would still have the other one. The healthy one. But now I didn't.

Renu sent me a list of articles about surgeons who were striving to do partial adrenalectomies whenever possible. If Dr. Blevins was skeptical when I forwarded an email from my spiritual teacher, he didn't show it. He responded with a respectful but noncommittal, "Well, that's something to investigate."

"I've been doing a lot of research," I said. "I don't want to lose the adrenal gland I have left. I need to see if I'm a candidate for the partial adrenalectomy."

"Partial adrenalectomy can be done in some cases," he said, "but it's a long shot."

"I've read the studies. I know there's a possibility of having to go back for another surgery, but the recurrence rate is relatively low. It's more than worth the risk."

He turned to his computer and tapped at the keyboard.

"Something else I need to say," I hedged. "I appreciate everything you've done for me, and I know that what happened is in no way your fault, but I need to move on to a different endocrinologist."

It was awkward. We'd been through so much together in such a short time. It felt like breaking up with someone, and I hated to lose this trusted ally. Dr. Blevins was the one who diagnosed this problem while other physicians ignored it. I wasn't even his patient at the time. He'd reached out, above and beyond his own obligations, and when everything went wrong, he took the heat for it. He listened as Eduardo and my parents unloaded the rage that rightly belonged in Dr. Humano's lap. I thought it was very brave and manly of him.

"I'm truly grateful for everything you've done to help me," I said, "but I need to distance myself from this whole experience with Dr. Humano."

"Of course," he said. "I completely understand. I do hope you'll let me know how it goes."

"I will. Thank you."

He nodded, thinking for a moment. "My son is interning with a well-known endocrinologist at MD Anderson Cancer Center in Houston. One of the top researchers. It may be difficult to get an appointment, but he might be able to connect you with a surgeon willing to try the partial adrenalectomy."

It made me smile to hear that his son was following in his footsteps, and I was glad to have him make one last call on my behalf. I was in no position to turn down a good connection now.

I spent the next day making a dress for Paty. This was something I'd never done before, but I wanted to do something with my hands, something creative that had nothing to do with adrenal glands or hormones or amber bottles of medication. Wandering between the rows of brightly colored bolts at the fabric store, I realized that since that terrible moment in the parking lot at Red Lobster, I had not left the house for anything other than doctor appointments. I chose a crisp white cotton with little blue triangles, some yellow damask, and a few yards of white lace and spent a long, pleasant day piecing together the full skirt and fitted bodice.

Blanca had made tostadas, and the kids were excited to tell us about their day. Eddie was up to his elbows in beans, Paty was excited about her new dress, and Lore was delivering an impassioned monologue about something that had happened at gymnastics. I looked across the table at Eduardo, and for a moment, we were just us, just a family with nothing haunting or hanging over us.

My phone buzzed next to my elbow. Before all this, Eduardo and I always left our phones in the other room during dinner. These days, we laid them on the table like part of the flatware. Butter knife, salad fork, cell phone.

"It's Dr. Blevins," I said.

Eduardo nodded. We'd opted not to tell the children anything just yet, so I left the table to take it in the next room. As I moved through the hallway, I heard Eduardo telling the kids to eat their veggies and not just the cheese. Life goes on.

"I was able to get you an appointment with Dr. Jimenez at MD Anderson," said Dr. Blevins. "No guarantees, but if anyone can get you on the docket for the partial adrenalectomy, it's him."

Two days later, Eduardo and I drove to Houston, hoping for the best. He was quiet for most of the three-hour drive, his gaze locked on the road ahead of us. The long drive from Austin to Houston begins and ends with hectic city traffic, but in between, there's two hours of Hill Country, cattle land, and vast meadows full of wild flowers. You have to slow down as you pass through Wyldwood, La Grange, Smithville, and several other small towns—all notorious speed traps—so we became familiar with all the quaint courthouses, taverns, and abandoned farmhouses. We had plenty of time to talk and plenty of time to not talk. Plenty of time to be in my head.

We'd spoken very little about the lawsuit since the initial blowup, but I knew it was on his mind. I knew it was a test of will for him to resist bringing it up, and I appreciated his effort to give me space and time to think about it on my own. In some ways, I found the lawsuit more daunting than a second surgery. I wanted to do the right thing, and I honestly didn't know what that would be.

"It's not about the money," people kept saying. "You don't want him to hurt anyone else, do you?" And of course, I didn't want that. It weighed on me heavily. Eduardo and I lived an extraordinary life, and we were able to provide extraordinary lives for our children. I'd always felt it was my duty to "pay it forward." Perhaps my adrenal gland had been taken so I would have the capacity to give something else. Was it my responsibility to fight this battle on behalf of another patient who didn't have the resources to fight for herself?

"How could he get it wrong like that?" I said. "I'll never understand."

Eduardo shook his head, his jaw tightly squared.

"I keep looking at the pathology report. Three times, it says *right*. Only that very last line says *left*. And if he had looked at the scans—I mean, obviously . . ."

"Apparently, he missed the day they covered left and right in medical school."

"There are exactly 237 words in the pathologist's report. Paty could have read it! How did he not read it? *Why* would he not read it?"

My heart raced. The skin around the healed incisions felt hot and alive with spiders. I felt all the clammy physical effects of the anger I'd been avoiding. Suddenly it was all coming to the surface.

"He was so proud of himself. So impressed with his tiny little incisions. *Oh, you won't even see the scar.* He got the job done in no time at all. In and out. No big deal. No question, he is a wonderful surgeon. But what good is your perfectly pretty surgery and your smooth bedside manner if you take out the *wrong organ*? I'd rather have my belly look like I'd been mauled by a tiger—as long as I could live my life."

Eduardo let me exhaust myself, venting all the rage my loved ones had let rip the moment they learned the truth. Eventually, I arrived at the place where they'd started.

"I want to sue him," I said.

"You're sure?"

"Yes."

"Okay." Eduardo squeezed my hand. "I know it's hard for you. It's not your nature. You want to believe the best about everybody. You want everyone to be happy. You have a kind heart. That's one of the things I love about you."

"I hate the whole idea, but I feel like I have to do it."

"We'll do it together."

We wove through the downtown traffic to the medical neighborhood in Houston. MD Anderson Cancer Center is like an industrial complex, a sprawling maze of towering office and hospital buildings, parking decks, lab and research facilities, hotels, restaurants, skywalks, and its own transit system. In the lobby of the endocrinology building, Eduardo and I met up with my parents, who'd flown in from Mexico. By now I was used to the intake procedure, but this was more like an assembly line.

I had all my paperwork prepared, including a lengthy questionnaire that asked probing questions like, "Do you think about death?" I doubted that anyone has ever walked into a cancer center without thinking about death, but I didn't want to open a can of worms, so I marked the "no" column. To be honest, there were many times when I thought my family might be better off if I just disappeared. That's the sort of ugly whispers that come with depression. But with the harsh truth had come a great sense of relief and new hope. I wasn't crazy. I wasn't losing my mind. I couldn't change what happened, but I could make it better.

Before we went to Dr. Jimenez's office, I went to phlebotomy to have my blood drawn, and the procedure was done in a large open space where patients were lined up, one after another, waiting for our number to be called. Looking around me, I saw a hundred stories just like mine. Not the same diagnosis. Something deeper than that. I saw eyes haunted by pain, frustration, and fear. I saw families bound by love and determination. I saw people in the act of surviving, and I was one of them. One of the lucky ones. *Death is in this place*, I thought, *but so is hope*. As the nurse tied a tourniquet on my arm, I closed my eyes and envisioned that angelic white light, willing it to radiate throughout the room.

We found our way to the endocrinology department, a long trek through breezeways, corridors, elevators, and a bus connection. The nurse in Dr. Jimenez's office took my vitals and showed me to the exam room, which wasn't geared for the traditional Mexican family. There was only one chair next to the exam table with its white paper.

butcher paper, la voz whispered.

"Anything else you want the doctor to know?" the nurse asked, flipping through my paperwork. This is an important question, I've learned. Your response will set the tone for the appointment because it's the last thing the doctor sees before he opens the door. It tells him what mood you're in, what your priorities are, and how well you're able to articulate your situation. I wanted to convey that I was interested in facts, respectful of his time, and not freaking out.

I nutshelled it for her. "I had a tumor on my right adrenal gland. The surgeon accidentally removed the left adrenal gland. Since then, I've experienced a range of symptoms that severely compromised quality of life." I didn't spill out the whole tale of woe, and I purposely avoided the word *malpractice* and anything else that might sound adversarial. The nurse made her notes on my chart and posted it by the door.

"Dr. Jimenez will be in shortly," she said and pulled the door closed behind her.

Papi insisted on standing, offering Mami the chair, but she was too agitated to sit. Several minutes ticked by. No gentle knock on the door.

"I hope they haven't forgotten about us," Mami said.

"They haven't," I assured her.

"I'll just check." She couldn't resist cracking the door to peek down the hallway. "I'll just leave this open a little so they know we're here."

Eduardo and I exchanged a glance, and he smiled and shrugged. I suppose he's seen me at enough appointments with my children to know I tend to be just as busily vigilant as Mami. And looking back, I see that I benefited from her example. It is important to insist on being seen, to make sure you're not forgotten. My God, if anyone has learned the importance of vigilance—how imperative it is to question, define, and demand the care you need—it would be me and my family. Acting like an obedient little mouse is not a sign of respect; it's a sign of intimidation. How could that possibly be healthy? The *good patient*, I've learned from Mami's example and from my own experience, is the patient who is well informed, proactive, and plainspoken. If your doctor prefers a patient who is uninformed, subservient, and too timid to speak, you need a different doctor.

"Hola, Señora Lorena!"

Dr. Jimenez entered the room like a cool breeze, sharp-dressed in a well-tailored suit. His hair was slicked back, not a strand out of place. He looked like he should be guest-starring on *Grey's Anatomy*, styled for drama. Mami arched an eyebrow at me. She didn't even have to say a word about the sweats and easygoing tunic I'd chosen to wear. She was wearing her crisis management uniform—crisp black pants and a pink blouse—in which she could smoothly attend a book club meeting, ER backstage, or Wednesday night mass.

When he greeted Eduardo and my parents, he offered his hand with the palm facing down, like the pope offering his ring for a kiss, but his smile was genuine, and he spoke Spanish to us, which

I found refreshing. A lot of Hispanic people avoid using Spanish in conversation with strangers, eager to clear away any question of how well assimilated they are to life in the United States.

"Tell me what's happening," he said.

Every time I had to retell the story, I felt a flush of anger rising like a warm tide. He listened with an expression of empathy, but there was no shock or alarm in his face. He was the most astonishingly pretty doctor I've ever seen. Throughout the conversation, he was very much the scientist, measured and precise when questioning or answering. The only small talk was to set me at ease while he conducted the exam.

"So. You're from Mexico?"

"Yes. Monterrey."

He touched my puffy neck below my chin. "How long have you had this dark patch?"

"A few weeks."

"What about this mole?" He touched my shoulder.

"Years. I've had it checked."

"I specialize in endocrine neoplasia and hormonal disorders," he said. "With adrenal complications, we sometimes see dark pigmentation." He looked me over, checking my eyelids, my fingertips, and the back of my neck. "No sign of cancer here."

"What's our next step?" I asked.

"I'd like you to speak with our surgeon, Dr. Perrier," he said. "It's difficult to get an appointment with Dr. Perrier. I'll make a call and see what I can do."

"So she could see Lorena today?" said Mami.

"Well." He smiled patiently. "Probably not. She's very busy. Maybe next week."

He sat down to make a note of this on the computer, and when he crossed his legs, Mami said, "What beautiful shoes you have, Dr. Jimenez. Where did you get them?"

I looked at her, incredulous. Like all mothers and daughters, we have our unspoken language, so I know she heard me loud and clear—*Seriously, Mami?*—but the doctor's eyes lit up.

"They were a gift," he said. "Made in Spain."

"Beautiful craftsmanship, Dr. Jimenez. Would you mind sharing the shoemaker's name with me?"

"Certainly."

He wrote out the information for her, and Mami engaged him in a brief but animated conversation about the process.

"I'll make a call," said Dr. Jimenez. "It's a long drive. Maybe they could work Lorena in this afternoon."

Mami thanked him, and we left with another round of warm, pope-style handshakes.

"Another brilliant mind," said Papi as we stood in line at the cafeteria. "Latin American talent seeping out to the US where talents like his shine." It made him frustrated with Latin American governments.

After lunch, we were still waiting for the doctor to call. Exhausted, I wanted to go to a hotel and take a nap, but Eduardo decided we should go to the boutique and buy a tie for Dr. Jimenez.

"A tie?" I said.

"We want him to like you," said my husband, and I laughed.

"If you say so."

"Hey, go ahead and mock. Relationship-building matters."

While we were out shopping for the tie, I got a message confirming the appointment at three. Gotta respect Mami's laser-true instincts. She'd clearly scored some points.

"Good call on the tie," I told Eduardo. We bought one that reflected both good taste and profound gratitude.

Mami and Papi met us in the reception area, and Dr. Perrier met us in the exam room a few minutes later, a petite blonde in a classy pencil skirt, pearl earrings, and Chanel pumps.

"Thank you so much for seeing me," I said. "I appreciate your time."

"My pleasure. Dr. Jimenez told me your story. Unbelievable. I'm so sorry this is happening to you." She spoke with a soft Southern lilt, but her manner was confident and authoritative. "I looked at the scans. The tumor is as plain as a blueberry in a pancake, and as a rule, I don't remove anything without touching it first."

"Is Lorena a candidate for the partial adrenalectomy?" Mami asked.

"I can't make any promises," said Dr. Perrier. "Partials are challenging due to the number of blood vessels in that tiny area. I need to study the tumor placement."

I liked Dr. Perrier. She was old enough to be experienced, young enough to not be stuck in old ways of doing things. She talked about forming a strategy very unlike the "this is how we do it" approach to the first surgery. Dr. Perrier was very specific about when and where and how she was willing to try the delicate procedure. It had to be on a Wednesday. She wanted specific OR staff involved. I would have to be patient while she collected the right team and did the required homework, but that was fine with me. If a concert pianist is to perform at her best, the piano has to be tuned, the acoustics have to be just right, and the pianist herself has to be at her best.

"You need to know," she said, "we may have to remove the whole thing, but if there's even a small chance of saving the adrenal gland, I will fight for it."

Later, after visiting with a cardiologist who wore a lilac bow tie, Eduardo and I made our way through the massive parking deck.

"Strange doctors," he said.

"Definitely the most stylish doctors I've ever been poked and prodded by," I said. "But I like them."

"I do, too. I think the day went well."

"We'll see," I said. I'm an optimist and always will be, but my optimism had been bruised. I felt the need to brace it with a realistic management of expectations.

I wondered, if I'd been given the choice between her and Dr. Humano, what would I have said? Would I have been willing to wait for the concert pianist? Would I have slowed down long enough to think about it? Old-school conformity is comforting, and Dr. Humano spoke in fatherly absolutes that reassured me, talking about the superiority of the laparoscopic technique and the thousands of surgeries he'd sailed through. I trusted him. I never questioned.

It's nice to think that the physician who holds your life in his hands never makes mistakes. We place doctors on this pedestal of infallibility, and I'm sure some of them enjoy it, but it's a fairy tale we're telling ourselves in order to not be terrified. Maybe it's better to go in with a healthy amount of fear. Maybe when you see a doctor as human, the doctor is more likely to see you as human, too.

thirteen

We returned to South Padre so the kids could play out the remainder of their summer break on the beach. I was grateful to have our beach place to retreat to as we counted down the days. I hoped that being in this heavenly place would make the time go by more quickly. This summer seemed to have gone on for an entire lifetime; so much had changed since June, when this tumor was diagnosed. The first surgery took place almost immediately, and I gave myself only two weeks to recover before I went on vacation for two miserable weeks and then took the kids to South Padre to be with my family. It was mid-July when I passed out in the parking lot at Red Lobster and learned the horrible truth of my situation. The second adrenal surgery was scheduled to take place at the end of September, a seemingly endless month after our first meeting with Dr. Perrier.

The sun was due to rise at 7:13 a.m. that day. Other than that, I was not counting on anything. I went into the first surgery completely confident that all my problems would be resolved within a few days. Now, after eight weeks of chaos and confusion, I faced thirty-one days of waiting, in which I would have to sit here, hoping for the best, preparing for the worst, and trying to manage the symptoms of my condition. It was like trying to balance a basket of tennis balls on my head. Turning on a light might trigger a migraine. The honk of a car horn might set off a cascade of heart palpitations. If I found a comfortable position to sleep in, I was afraid to move, knowing I might be jolted awake with searing knots in my calves and feet.

One night during our first week back at the beach, I woke up shaking, my heart and lungs gripped by an invisible fist. I tried to slow my breathing, focusing my eyes on a painting that I loved—an abstract landscape with blue mountains and white cliffs between a red sky and green river valley. Since acquiring this painting years earlier, I'd spent hours looking at it, thinking, *Here is beauty. Here is balance.* But now the colors shifted and began to spin, and then the room began reeling around me. I gripped the edge of the bed as the floor pitched and swelled like the waves outside. I placed the palm of my hand on the nightstand. The sensation of cool marble against my feverish skin helped me center myself. I watched the painting return to its original composition.

Over the next few weeks, every time I woke up like this, I used this painting as my reality check as I worked out whether I was dreaming or awake or somewhere in between. Sometimes it took a while, but I knew it would eventually return to itself, and then I'd feel safe standing up.

I tried to surround myself with positive thoughts and energy, posting motivational quotes here and there. Some were store-bought canvas prints with bold Impact font: *My life is full of love.* Others were handmade with free-spirited script on an ombré background: *I choose happiness.* I found a letter—calligraphy on white canvas—and cried as I installed it on the wall in Lore and Paty's room. It was an optimistic love letter expressing belief in the best possible future for them along with the gratitude I felt every time I looked at their sweet faces. I wanted them to know that I was there, that I would not just disappear.

Lore and Paty wanted to spend every waking moment playing in the sand and water, of course, and Eddie wanted to be wherever his big sisters were, so I spent a lot of time sitting in the shade, listening to them splash and chase one another. When Roby was pregnant, waiting out the agonizing weeks before she could have her cancer surgery, my sisters and I sat with Mami in this very spot. We never left Roby alone. Someone was always there. Now here we were again, and it was my turn to wait and be watched over. The Gulf of Mexico was deep and beautiful, even when it was troubled. It was constantly in motion, constantly changing, but always the same, always there for me. Like my family.

The ongoing discussion of the lawsuit was always in the background. Our attorney, who is also a good friend, connected us to an elite Houston law firm where one of the attorneys was actually an adrenal surgeon. When Eduardo shared this news with my parents and siblings, everyone was thrilled. What astonishingly good luck, they all agreed, and I tried to be glad, but the whole thing went against my grain.

"This is good news," Eduardo said.

"I have no adrenaline," I reminded him. (My friend Malia made me laugh about that. "Does that mean you could fall asleep on a roller coaster?")

Eduardo and my father had enough adrenaline to make up for my lack of it. All that rage had settled to grim determination fueled by love for me, anger at this man who'd hurt me, and a strong dose of testosterone. I joked about it, but looking back, I wonder if my lack of adrenaline allowed me to compartmentalize and consider all this differently. My emotions rose and fell, spiking and bottoming out, and it was probably healthy for me to experience the full spectrum. Anger can be a cleansing fire. Sorrow is really a form of gratitude, when you think about it. Even self-pity has its place. For me, the most terrifying moments were the times when I felt nothing.

Lore's birthday was coming up, and I had not prepared anything. I kept telling myself, "Tomorrow. I'll take care of it tomorrow, for sure." But the days slipped by, one after another. At the last minute, I sent Blanca to the store.

"Could you please get a cake," I said, "and . . . I guess . . . whatever looks nice."

Overwhelmed with fatigue and nausea, I had to lie down and nap. When I dragged myself down to join the party, I found the garish, carnival-themed cake in the kitchen and my family already gathered in the game room. All the cousins were tearing around, stoked with sugar, batting red-and-yellow balloons. I felt like an awkward guest at the party I should have designed and hosted. The cake and decorations should have been unique, special to Lore's unique personality, not hastily store-bought from the shelf. She was happy enough, dressed in a pink dress with red polka dots.

"Here's Mama!" Eduardo was happy to see me. "*Mi amorcito*, you're just in time for pictures."

I posed with Lore next to the carnival cake, a plastic smile on my face, and I managed to stay long enough to see her blow out the candles, but the smell of the sugary icing and melted wax turned my stomach. I had to dash to the bathroom to throw up, and then I went outside to sit on the sand, feeling desolate, furious at myself for failing such a simple task as a child's birthday party. I have to wonder now: Why was it so easy for me to hate myself and so impossible for me to hate the surgeon who'd robbed my children of their mother?

My sense of time during those weeks was warped and undependable. An hour might be the blink of an eye or a long, arduous voyage. Looking back, I have only a few hazy memories of those days on the beach, as if my brain refused to form the chemical bonds that keep things in your mental filing cabinet. I know I got up in the morning and helped the kids into their swimsuits. I poured cereal and orange juice and put on a sundress and sandals. The mechanics of the morning pulled me along until I was sitting on a sling chair between my sisters, and then I could give in to the exhausting drag of gravity.

One afternoon, Paty danced over to me and said, "Mom, can we make you a mermaid?"

"Yes, Mama!" Lore tugged on my hand. "Lie down and don't move."

Roby and Mami clucked, "Lorena, your dress will be full of sand," but I laughed and stretched out on the ground. The girls set to work, piling sand to cocoon me from the waist down. I closed my eyes and listened to them giggle as they shaped a graceful tail down by my feet. It felt good to lie still, weighed down by cool sand as they transformed me. I became a mermaid, a creature in between. I stayed as long as I could, suspended between earth and water, but eventually I had to get up and brush myself off.

The closest condo was Mami's, so I went inside and took a shower in her bathroom. I rinsed all the sand from my body, wrapped myself in a bath sheet, and padded barefoot down the hall to the room where my grandmother had stayed when she came to visit. It was clean and silent. Mami had not changed anything since Abuela died.

"Abuela," I said softly, "I wish you were here."

I took a quartz crystal from the night table and held it in my hands, certain that my grandmother had held it in her hands when she was here. I lay down on the bed where she slept and dreamed, craving her guidance, needing to feel her presence. What would she have told me to do? The right thing, certainly, for the right reason. But what did that mean?

Cards, emails, gifts, and texts came to me from friends and family all over the world, expressing love and encouraging me to stay strong. Word travels fast when there's a ghastly plot twist in the story. I appreciated the prayers and well wishes, but in almost all the correspondence was the common theme: "I hope you sue that bastard for everything he's worth." Some people seemed to think I'd won the lottery and should take some pleasure in this windfall coming my way. Mostly, though, there was an assumption that I would—and should—do as much damage as possible to this person who had damaged me. They called this "justice," but to me, it sounded like revenge, and I didn't want that.

For me, the only upside of the lawsuit was for some good to come out of it: some new understanding, some change in the status quo that contributed to this situation. I needed to believe that some higher purpose could be served by all this, because if it wasn't, then the landscape of my life had been razed for nothing but a stupid, random blunder, and the thought of that was beyond unbearable. It was infuriating. It was *infuriating* that a tumor the size of a garbanzo bean went undiagnosed for so many months despite its devastating impact. It was *infuriating* that when I finally got someone to pay attention to me, he couldn't be troubled to look at the scan before he cut into my body. When I allowed myself to think about it, rising anger felt like a tight collar around my neck. I feared the physical and emotional fallout that came with anger. I longed for the peace that would come with forgiveness, and at first, I didn't see how anger and forgiveness could coexist.

Deeply ingrained in me was a well-behaved woman who'd been taught to defer. All good girls know that anger isn't ladylike, Christian, or socially acceptable. "Forgive and forget," we're told. And this is fine for the everyday slights that come our way. Life with a family like mine is full of opportunities for little rifts, if you allow it, and I never did. Let it go. Get over it.

But this was above and beyond that. This situation was so egregious, there was no letting go, no moving on, no "forgive and forget." I live with the consequences every day. It would be ridiculous—and hypocritical—to pretend that I never get angry about it. The truth is, trying to forgive without anger is like trying to bake bread without yeast. The sincerity of your forgiveness is directly proportional to the sincerity of your anger. If you deny your anger, your forgiveness is lip service, an empty prayer. And that anger doesn't just evaporate. It has to go somewhere, so it goes inward, to the heart of you.

It took me a while to understand this. All I could do during those waiting weeks was cycle through it all again and again, like a spiral staircase—around and around you go until, eventually, you reach higher ground.

This anger was my right. I'd paid a terrible price for it. It was mine to hold on to or let go of, however and whenever I chose to. For the moment, I embraced it. Every once in a while, I had to allow myself to rage, weep, and swear, which was not easy for me. A friend advised me to go somewhere and scream, but where does one go to scream when one has little children? Not the car, not the closet, not the beach. Ultimately, I made good use of the shower, cranking it on as hard as it would go, howling up into the jets of hot water. I began to see that the physical and emotional fallout of embracing my anger was less devastating than the physical and emotional fallout of repressing it. Instead of directing it inward to choke me, I let it blaze outward and energize me.

fourteen

In September, we went home to Austin and settled into the routine of a new school year. It felt good to move forward with life and not feel like everything was on hold. I'd invested all my hope and confidence in that first surgery as a one-stop fix. Get in, get out, get on with your life. Going into the second surgery, I had to accept that this was my life now; the second surgery was just one step in managing a lifelong chronic health issue.

The topic of the lawsuit was always hanging in the air, but I refused to be nudged into anything I wasn't ready for.

"I can't make any decisions until I get past this second surgery," I told Eduardo. "I just want this thing out of me. Then we can see how we feel about the next step. Until I wake up, we have no way of knowing if I'll have even a fragment of an adrenal gland."

He agreed that this was a wise approach, and he was glad to hear that I wanted my family with me this time. No stubborn desire to go through surgery by myself. This time, taking ownership of the surgery meant accepting the unknowns and accepting help. This surgery would be far more invasive than the first procedure. Entering from my abdomen would not be possible, another bridge burned.

"To avoid the site of the recent surgery," said Dr. Perrier, "I'll have to go in through your back under your ribs, so there is some risk of nerve damage, and I may have to make a larger incision."

Instead of a few tiny "bikini-friendly" incisions, this time I really could end up looking like the magician's assistant. There would be a lot more deep tissue involved and a longer recovery process. I would have to swallow my pride and let my family help me through the aftermath—whatever that might be.

Instead of nodding and smiling through a quick summary of the procedure, I asked Dr. Perrier endless questions—how, exactly, do you do this or that—and took copious notes as she laid out the specifics. The big unknown was whether I'd wake up with a scrap of an adrenal gland or no adrenal function at all.

"No promises," she said, "but I'll do my best."

I spent time in my grateful corner, which expanded to include cards, letters, and small works of art. When I closed my eyes to meditate, I saw myself at the center of a swirling galaxy of souls— my people, my family. My connection to them is unlimited by time, space, or even death. When Tía Paty gave me a white-and-gold crucifix that had belonged to her mother, she told me, "My mother said it made miracles. Now I pray for a miracle for you." She placed it in my hands, and I felt her miraculous love.

Before I left for Houston, my friends gathered at my home, the way you would gather for a baby or bridal shower. (A surgery shower! If this is not a thing, it should be.) They gave me a collection of polished stones, each one etched with a word of blessing— *peace, strength, grace*—and presented me with a *ramillete espiritual* ("spiritual bouquet") of hopes and prayers. The next morning I placed the stones in my suitcase with all my comfort needs and necessities and climbed into the car with Eduardo, Mami, and Papi.

Before the surgery, I had three days of pre-op tests, scans, and blood work. Between appointments, I napped or stared vacantly at the television. My mother tried to lift my spirits by taking me shopping, but it was crowded, and the faces of the shoppers bustling by warped and fuzzed. Feeling myself becoming disoriented, I stared down at their feet instead. It was like the parade of feet in the wedding carpet film. Constant motion. Every direction. Each person going their own direction. I wrapped my arms around myself and said, "Mami, I need to get out of here."

She didn't chide or cheer me on or tell me I was being too sensitive. She took my arm, steered me to the nearest exit, and pushed through the revolving doors. I was grateful to be out in the autumn air, grateful to have Mami at my side, and grateful to know I had nothing else to do that day but crawl into my bed back at the hotel.

The next day, my friend Luz arrived from Mexico City. It was a wonderful surprise, and I took it as a good omen. Luz means "light," and she definitely brought light and lightness with her. I hadn't seen her in fifteen years, but we were inseparable when we were growing up and had the kind of friendship that always picks up again right where it left off, no matter how much time has flown by. I was so grateful for her calm presence now, anchoring me to the energized young woman I was before all this trouble. And a crazy thing happened when we sat down for dinner in the hotel restaurant that night. Seated at the table next to us was an old friend from Monterrey.

"Lorena!" She stood up and waved. "I thought that was you."

"Oh . . . Maria!" It took me a moment to recognize her. I'd always known her with long dark hair, and now she was sporting a cute blonde bob. When I went to give her a hug, I realized it was a wig.

"You remember my mother," she said, "and this is my new friend Amla and her mother. We met here at MD Anderson."

The mothers and daughters joined our table, and we all finished dinner together, exchanging stories and coping strategies.

Amla's mother shared a great tip: There was a hotel nearby where you could get a hospital bed in the room.

"God bless you tomorrow," said Maria's mother. She held both my hands between her own, and I could feel her grandmotherly prayers.

When Luz and I parted ways in the hallway, she said, "Sleep tight. I'll be there in the morning with your mom."

Eduardo and I lay awake most of the night, huddled close and breathing softly, each of us trying not to disturb the other, neither of us really sleeping. I ran through the schedule in my mind. I'd prepared as carefully as if I were reciting for an exam, thinking of everything. I had warmer socks this time and a shirt I could wear without a bra. More important, I was showing up with an awareness I lacked before. I made the conscious decision to be present in each moment. I wasn't just wishing it would be over. I was focusing all my intentions on the room I was in right now, never getting ahead of myself. Instead of attaching myself to one specific outcome, I opened myself to the best versions of all outcomes by seeing the best version of myself in whatever scenario lay ahead.

I was conscious of every detail. When Eduardo and I sat down with the clipboard to fill out the final paperwork, I immediately noticed the line where the surgery was described.

"Eduardo, look." I pointed to it with the tip of the pen. "It says 'removal of the right adrenal.' That's only the worst-case scenario."

"That's not right," he agreed. "Sit tight. I'll take care of it."

He took the paperwork back to the nurse and spoke to her quietly but firmly. "Excuse me. This should say 'partial removal of right adrenal.'"

She smiled and said, "Oh, no worries. The doctor knows."

Eduardo smiled back. "Lorena will not sign this until it says *partial.*"

"Sir, it would take like thirty minutes for us to—"

"We'll wait."

"Okay. Have a seat. I'll let you know when it's ready." She puffed an exasperated sigh, but a little while later, she came back with the amended paperwork, still warm from the laser printer. "Everything okay now?"

I skimmed to the description: *PARTIAL REMOVAL of right adrenal.*

"Yes," I said. "Thank you."

I knew the drill. Vitals, gown up, start the IV, meet the team. The anesthesiologist started the numbing cocktail. Mami leaned in close to my ear and whispered, "*Hijita*," a term of endearment that expressed motherly love for her little daughter. She always leaves me with that small blessing. "*Hijita*, I'll be praying." She left to sit with Papi, who was already pacing in the waiting room, fidgeting with his hands in his pockets, asking people if they needed coffee.

Eduardo kissed my forehead and said, "See you soon."

Petite Dr. Perrier looked even smaller in her scrubs and flat, paper-sheathed surgical shoes, but her presence was big, her voice confident.

She bent over the gurney. "Ready, Lorena?"

"I'm ready."

Instead of focusing the white light on myself, I let it flow through me to each and every corner of the room. White light on the surgeon's hands. White light on the instruments laid out on the steel table. White light on the OR nurses as they came and went, on the monitors, computer screens, and spotlights. White light on the ceiling and swinging doors, to the hallway, to the rooftop, and to the wild blue autumn sky. I slipped out of time, out of place, and then—in what seemed like less than a moment—I became aware of soft voices and the steady *pip pip* of a heart monitor.

Coming out of the first surgery, my first thought was, *It's over.*

Coming out of the second surgery, my first thought was, *It begins.*

I took inventory. Toes. Knees. Torso. Arms. Through the haze of painkillers, I surveyed the injury to my body. I felt impaled, as if a spear had gone through me.

"Lorena?" It was a nurse. I must be in the recovery room. "Lorena, how are you feeling?"

"Sleepy."

"That's to be expected."

"Did everything go okay?"

"The doctor will be here shortly."

I drifted off again and resurfaced after what felt like a thousand years. I smelled the clean, mellow scent of Eduardo's cologne and felt the warmth of his hand on my face.

"You're a champion," he said.

A little while later, Dr. Perrier arrived, back in her chic pencil skirt, pearls, and Chanel heels.

"The partial was successful," she said. "We were able to save about 40 percent of your adrenal gland."

It would be a balancing act, monitoring my blood work, taking precautions, and adjusting medications for the rest of my life. My adrenal function was still severely compromised, but it meant so much to me that she'd fought for—and won—this small victory.

In the days that followed, I allowed myself to sink into the muffled blur of morphine and sleep. I was vaguely aware of the process to disconnect me from the monitors, catheter, and IV. My family and friends came and went with flowers, prayers, and loving words. My brother sent me a letter from Monterrey, and my unconditionally loving friend, Kristy, read it to me, moved to tears by his big brotherly love. So many people came to see me that the charge nurse had to set a limit on my visitors, which was all right.

I needed a silent moment to relocate my feet, figure out how to use the bathroom, and process this new shock to my system.

Surgery, as I said, is violent, even when the results are everything you hoped for. You have to honor that and give the experience due respect. I did that this time, instead of fixating and rushing toward some false ideal of "okay" that was never going to happen. This time, I allowed myself to trust, to fall back into the arms of people who were there to care for me. I allowed both tears and laughter as needed, allowed grief and relief to coexist. I never scolded myself about feeling the wrong feelings or thinking the wrong thoughts.

I was acutely self-aware, never ignoring or shaming myself as my body struggled to realign itself. The symptoms of my adrenal mayhem had terrorized me after the first surgery. Every migraine, every fainting spell, every heart palpitation, even that wretched little *la voz* was my body screaming at me, "*This is wrong! This is wrong!*" Instead of listening to my body, I listened to Dr. Humano tell me, "You're fine." Now I listened to the higher wisdom of my body and let it guide me. I still wasn't fine, but I saw new symptoms as benevolent couriers, code-talkers translating the secret language of my endocrine system. Instead of muzzling symptoms with drugs, I allowed them to guide me and my new endocrinologist toward actual solutions.

My friend Anne was undergoing aggressive treatment for cancer that summer, and because I had my patient bracelet, I was able to go and visit her. She had to be isolated, so we looked at each other through a thick glass window and spoke to each other on old-fashioned telephones, the way you see people do in the movies when one of them is in jail. Sometimes, there was not much need for the telephones. Sometimes there was nothing to say; we just pressed our hands to the glass, palm to palm, and let ourselves be understood. When we see each other in the real world now, we find that we still communicate in the unspoken language of that shared experience.

I was released from the hospital four days after the surgery. Rather than attempt to travel home, I moved to the hotel with the hospital bed. There was a bit of a false start; I had to go back to the hospital almost immediately because of cardiomegaly. (My heart was enlarged due to all those months of high blood pressure.) *Here we go again*, I thought. It was discouraging, but after a few days, I was back in the hotel, surrounded by my family.

My brother arrived, bringing canvas bags of organic groceries and goodies. He and my father tinkered with the settings on the hospital bed to find the exact settings where I would be most comfortable and remained on call for any errands that needed to be run. Roby arrived with magazines and music and lots of little sister ridiculousness to make me laugh. My mother stood constant vigil, anticipating every need, making sure I had food before I was hungry, water before I was thirsty, and a shawl before I caught a chill. She helped me make sense of my curly hair, massaged my feet, and rubbed lotion into my dry elbows. When I had to use the bathroom, she waited outside the door and then came in to help me with—well, you know. Hygiene issues.

"Mami," I said, "I'm so sorry you have to do this."

"Do what?"

"Wipe my bottom. This isn't exactly the highlight of anyone's day."

"This isn't the first time I wiped your bottom. I'm the one who changed your diapers, don't forget." She helped me stand, steadying me as I shuffled back to my bed. "I don't feel any different about it now. You're still my baby, *hijita*."

Most uplifting, most healing, were the quiet hours when Eduardo lay beside me on the bed and our children played in a broad square of sunlight from the sliding balcony doors. Sometimes we watched movies and listened to music. Sometimes Lore and Paty danced and sang for us. They staged fashion shows and presented educational programs featuring poetry, art, Mandarin vocabulary, and other things they learned in school. Eddie joined in, clowning around, making me laugh until I had to hold a pillow against my aching midsection. They never complained that they were bored or bothered about being cooped up in a hotel room. They were just overjoyed to have me back, closer to being myself than I'd been in a long, long time. They craved the closeness they'd missed during all those months when I was thickly encased in misery and incapable of true closeness. It may sound strange, but those quiet weeks with my family in that hotel room are among the happiest memories of my life.

When it was time to make the difficult drive back to Austin, my father went home ahead of us and engineered an ingenious system of ropes between the doors, windows, and furniture to help me stand up, sit down, and steady myself while the flesh and muscle tissue in my poor torso continued to knit itself back together. The network of ropes and handholds looked like a transit map with stops at all the places I needed to be: my bedroom, the bathroom, the kitchen, the front door, and a favorite chair by the window where I could read a book or watch the kids play in the swimming pool. Day by day, I got stronger. After two weeks, it was getting easier to pull myself up, and after a month, I was solid on my own two feet again. This is what recovery is, I suppose. You pull yourself up and move on. What a world of difference it makes when someone has gone ahead of you to rig a few strategic handholds.

If you've seen the movie *Coco* (and you must see it!), you've glimpsed the great importance of family in Mexican culture. My extended family is a sprawling, noisy, colorful mess at times, and of course, there are times when maybe it's not so helpful to have forty strong opinions coming at you all at once, but it's an extravagant luxury to be loved the way we love one another in my family. It's a privilege to be there for my sisters and cousins the way they were there for me. I aspire to be the matriarch my mother is and to someday be as courageous and wise as my father. I enjoy the idea that Eduardo and I will someday be the elders, as protective and fiercely loving as my aunts and uncles.

During my stay at MD Anderson, I saw so many people going through chemo alone except for the support of volunteers. These caregivers inspired me and reminded me of the caregiving component of my own soul, something I'd almost forgotten about during this dark, needy time. Thinking about them in the months and years that followed, I came to two conclusions. First, I would never again take for granted the bounty of my family's love. And second, I would someday find a way to care for strangers as if they were part of my family.

fifteen

Whoever you are, wherever you are as you read this, I promise, you are stronger than you think you are. And I promise, the thing you fear most is not the thing that requires your greatest strength. The life you rebuild and live after you slay your personal dragon—sustainable day-to-day existence—this is the challenge that tests your last grain of strength. Well-meaning people will tell you it's time to "get back to normal" or encourage you to find a "new normal"—but "normal" is a fairy tale. By definition, "normal" exists only as a comparison to what other people have. How can that be healthy—to be constantly comparing ourselves to others?

Three weeks after the second surgery, I studied my altered body in the mirror. The lingering swelling along with the nerve damage Dr. Perrier had warned me about left me with a lopsided silhouette. My belly button was strangely off center. (Definitely not normal.) I hated the weight I'd gained and wasn't eager to put myself out there at a social event, but in October, the Formula One Grand Prix was happening in Austin, and Eduardo was hosting a party. He would have understood if I'd opted out, but this was a big deal, an important social and business function, and I wanted to support him as I always have. I grew up watching my parents build their world together; my father would not be who and what he is without my mother. I wanted to be no less than that tower of strength for my husband.

Mami hired someone to come to do our hair and makeup at her house. When I arrived, she looked worried. "Are you sure you feel up to this?"

"No," I said, "but I'm doing it. It'll be fine."

When my face was on, I gritted my teeth and eased myself into shapewear and a cocktail dress. I've always been a person who loves to dress up. I love fashion as an art form and appreciate the skill it takes to craft hair and makeup. I love the look on Eduardo's face when he sees me done up and ready to take on the world with him. All that said, this was not a great moment for pageantry. It took all my will to force my swollen feet into the electric-blue heels that used to make me feel like Wonder Woman.

Mami looked me over and nodded. "You look lovely!"

I went to Lore and Paty's room to kiss the children good-night. I knew Eddie would be there, too, because even though he has his own room, he loves to camp out with his sisters, and his sisters love to have him. They all came running to hug me.

"Mommy, you look beautiful!"

I carefully bent forward and pressed kisses to the crowns of their heads. I would have loved to be in pj's, cuddling in with them to watch a movie, but when I went downstairs, there was Eduardo with that look on his face. Racing is one of his passions, and he's masterful at forging the partnerships that transform passions—like racing, motorcycles, and soccer—into major industry deals.

We arrived early at the Driskill, a spectacular hotel in downtown Austin. The band was doing a sound check, dancers were warming up, and the caterers were hustling to ready the bars and buffet tables. In the past, I would have been all up in these details, my eye on every knife and napkin. This was the first time I arrived at this sort of event having had nothing to do with the planning. Determined to make up for my absence, I was fully engaged. I mixed, mingled, and even danced a little, keeping my game face on from the moment the first guest arrived.

"I'm back!" I said, needing to declare it, even though I didn't really feel like I was back. I felt like I'd barely begun to climb the thousand-mile staircase to *back*. I was wearing a heart monitor under my cocktail dress. Instead of the busy work schedules, charity events, book club meetings, and lunch dates they were all chatting about, my calendar was filled with medical appointments, blood tests, and follow-up exams. But you know the old saying: "Fake it till you make it." That's what I was determined to do.

When friends and coworkers saw me, they said, "Your hair looks amazing!" or "I love your shoes!" or "You look so skinny in that dress!" They were being kind, I know, but one of the many lessons I've learned through hardship is that when you give a personal compliment, it's better to express something personal.

Your laughter is so contagious.

It's so much fun to be around you.

If someone compliments my hair, the next time I see them, I'm going to be self-conscious if my hair is out of control that day. We need to get past the idea that "Wow, you've lost weight!" is a compliment. Believe me, that one doesn't play well at MD Anderson where people are emaciated from chemo, and if you're already self-conscious about being overweight, it's painful to have your weight suddenly be at the center of the spotlight.

I love the wisdom you bring to a conversation.

You have such a good heart.

These are qualities that deserve to be celebrated, compliments that actually mean something lasting and contribute to the person's self-esteem, but for some reason, we've been trained to call out the superficial—clothes, shoes, hair—everything that's fleeting, unimportant, and far more changeable than anyone likes to think about.

Toward the end of the evening, I stepped out on the balcony, needing to breathe the cool night air. The loud music had given me a headache, and I was so ready to get out of my uncomfortable party clothes, but I was proud of the effort I'd made to be here for my husband. I was still standing.

In the first six or eight weeks that followed the surgery, Dr. Jimenez and Dr. Perrier were vigilant about following up with me, but once the surgery itself was accomplished, wound care tended to, healing of incisions verified, and a reasonable balance of adrenal function restored, they moved on. Through all this, Dr. Blevins checked on me and stayed on top of things, even though he was no longer my endocrinologist. I appreciated the way he remained in my life as a supportive friend who just happened to know everything there is to know about endocrinology, and eventually, I did go back to him. He practiced the highest standards in medicine and showed great integrity as a human being.

I had assembled a great team, and I knew I could make an appointment if I really needed to, but we were out of crisis mode now. Everyone, including me, expected that I could, should, and would get on with my life now and not require a lot of hand-holding. I found myself feeling very much alone with my cabinet full of pharmaceuticals and a severe case of separation anxiety. These doctors were my life raft when I desperately needed one. Now I would sink or swim on my own.

Reluctantly, I turned my attention to the lawsuit. Eduardo scheduled an appointment with the firm in Houston, which made sense because I would have to travel there regularly for surgical follow-up and appointments with the new endocrinologist. The highbrow Houston lawyers encouraged me to dive in and be aggressive, and everyone around me agreed that the most sensible course was to follow their lead.

I was certain of only one thing: I needed to take ownership of this lawsuit just as I was taking ownership of my health issues. Before I walked into a meeting with lawyers, I wanted to make sure that I was absolutely clear in my own mind about what I wanted and needed from this lawsuit. Eduardo and my parents would support me, whatever I needed to do, but these lawyers would have their own agenda—which was fine, as long as their agenda served mine.

"If it's just the money, it's not worth it," I said. "I don't need his money."

"What do you need?" asked Eduardo.

"Justice," I said, because that seemed like the right answer. "Justice" is what everyone else said they wanted for me, and it sounded like a noble goal, but I wondered: What does justice look like? An eye for an eye? A scale in perfect balance? A pendulum that swings to one extreme and then the other until it comes to a stop somewhere near center? No reparations or apologies could right this wrong. No biblical eye-for-an-eye balancing of the scales was even possible here. If I was ever to make peace with what happened to me, I'd have to find that balance within myself.

My father, more than anyone else in my life, has always been my moral compass, the one I look to for direction when I want to do the right thing, but I wanted him to give me the impartial advice he would give a stranger, and I didn't know if that was possible.

Loving someone changes everything.

"I want to do the right thing," I told him, "but this lawsuit doesn't feel right. I can't see any good coming from it, and I'd be devoting months—possibly years—to the effort of . . . of what? I don't even know what the goal is."

"You could do something good with the money," my father suggested. "I know there are great causes that mean a lot to you, and this money would mean a lot to them. You could start a foundation to fund research."

This idea did appeal to me, but along with my struggle to survive this thing, it felt like a burden I never signed up for and had no idea how to carry. I wanted some good to come from this, some form of healing equal to the hurt, but assigning a dollar value to what Dr. Humano had taken from me was beyond impossible. This was not only a part of my body, it was a part of my life, Eduardo's life, and the lives of our children.

"That's why we need to get creative," said the Houston lawyer. "Tell me everything. We have to paint a picture of the journey of your life." And by everything, he meant everything people want to think, not everything true. By marriage, he meant sex. By motherhood, he meant other people's idea of what a mother is supposed to be. By journey, he meant to have me play into some warped stereotype of the poor Mexican immigrant who comes to America to clean houses and dream an American dream. They were concerned that if a jury knew about the wealth and privilege in my life, they'd resent me the way some of my classmates did when we were kids.

"How is any of that relevant?" I asked. "Isn't this fairly obvious? He took the *wrong body part*. What more needs to be said?"

"If we want the maximum damages, we have to go beyond the malpractice itself. The more creative we get, the more money we can ask for."

They explained to me that money awarded would be paid by an insurance company, not by Dr. Humano, and any settlement we reached would likely depend on my willingness to sign a no-fault or nondisclosure agreement, which I wasn't willing to do. I wasn't willing to set aside my integrity. That's not how I was raised. The whole "get creative" conversation made me intensely uncomfortable, so our good friend suggested a local attorney with a folksier approach. We met with him at our home, and the conversation was very different in tone, but the bottom line was the same.

"How would this lawsuit make a difference?" I asked him.

"Difference?" He looked nonplussed. "Well, if it makes you feel better . . ."

"That's not what I mean. I'm trying to understand—will it make a *difference* in the system? Will this lawsuit impact the way doctors care for people? Will it change the way patients are heard? Will it change any aspect of surgical culture?"

He looked at me as if I were asking him to bring me the moon in a champagne flute. We discussed the possibility of going after Dr. Humano's medical license or insisting on a jury trial that would expose him to a lot of bad press. We could make him suffer, I was assured, but if there's any satisfaction to be found in the suffering of another person, it's a hollow satisfaction, a void within the soul. I wanted no part of that. "Getting even" is not justice; it's vengeance, and that felt toxic to me. What I really wanted—what I needed for my own healing—was to forgive. And I didn't know yet if that was possible.

I fully understood that forgiveness would be for my own good. I agree with what Anne Lamott wrote in the book *Traveling Mercies*: "Not forgiving is like drinking rat poison and then waiting for the rat to die." But to function as a true antidote to that poison, forgiveness must be *real*, and I wasn't there yet. Authentic forgiveness comes from a place of strength, and I had a long way to go before I could confidently say I felt strong again, physically or emotionally.

sixteen

That autumn rushed into the holiday season, and then the new year, and then another spring and summer. That year passed by me like a freight train, dominated by medical appointments, tests, scans, blood work, and the intricate balancing act of medications, hormones, and day-to-day life. I took classes and attended workshops on hormones, PTSD, and chronic pain. There were days when I genuinely questioned my ability to go on—questioned the very reason for working as hard as I had to work for a life that was only a shadow of the life I'd envisioned for myself.

Another autumn rushed in, and in November 2014, my hopes surged with the realization that I seemed to be regaining some sense of balance. I was able to curate and mount *Shaped in Mexico*, the London gallery exhibit I was working on when I was pregnant with Eddie. Eddie was now a robust toddler, running around and already kicking a soccer ball, which filled his father's heart with pride and joy. Lore and Paty were passing through that lovely preteen pony-leg stage, all knees and elbows. They spent the summer on the beach, two perfect mermaids splashing in the Gulf waters.

I sat down to write our Christmas letter to loved ones.

Dear family and friends,

Life sure is full of surprises. Last year was a tough one. When I was ready to conquer the world with my Shaped in Mexico *art project, I got very bad news. The surgeon removed the wrong adrenal gland. I still had the one with the tumor. My life started spiraling down in every way—health, emotions, spirituality. I couldn't help but ask God why me, why this. So instead of going to London, I was headed to MD Anderson hospital in Houston because they have one of the world's best surgeons for what I needed done.*

My conquering the world turned into conquering my health. All I wanted was to be well and to be back home with my husband and my kids. I lost any notion of what joy meant. I forgot why on earth I liked art. I lost me. I lost faith in doctors. I was furious deep inside. What was I doing wrong?

I decided to quiet down, to retreat a bit from everything to listen to myself. I embraced the new Lorena. I was not putting effort where I should have. I can't get my adrenal back, but I can get to know my new body, my limitations, my spirit. I listened to my body, my common sense, and let go of the past. Recognizing the humanity behind the surgeons, doctors, and nurses, I forgave what the surgeon had done. To be a good wife, mother, daughter, friend, boss, I have to be my new me.

There is something bigger than us. If we don't embrace life's difficulties as our teachers, we are not close to God. We are still wanting to be in control. But what you can really control and affect positively on others is how you dance through life.

So, one year later, I'm on my way back from my London edition of Shaped in Mexico. *It was a huge success. My heart is full and content. I did it. I have my life back, my beautiful—*

This was such bullshit, I couldn't even finish writing it, much less sign my name to it. I wanted it to be true. Desperately! But it wasn't.

Last year was a tough one? My God. Understatement of the century!

I was not putting effort where I should have. How about not putting effort into unwarranted self-blame?

I embraced the new Lorena. What about mourning the Lorena I had lost?

I forgave what the surgeon had done. Not. Even. Close.

Maya Angelou said: "You can't forgive without loving. And I don't mean sentimentality. I don't mean mush. I mean having enough courage to stand up and say, 'I forgive. I'm finished with it.'" That Christmas letter was pure mush, no matter how deeply I wanted to mean it.

I kept saying, "I have forgiven him," and every time I said it, I tried to mean it, wanting it to be true but knowing it wasn't. I felt like a phony, unable to live up to this standard I'd set for myself. Every time I was reminded of something else he'd taken from me, I felt newly wounded and freshly irate. Seeing a photograph of Eduardo and me on a motorcycle reminded me that I couldn't journey with him like that anymore. Planning a family ski trip reminded me that I would sit in the lodge reading a book. In the months and years that followed the botched surgery, I keep stumbling over loss after loss. Eventually, I was forced to confront the reality that forgiveness is an ongoing process. You don't just decide to forgive and then turn the page. That decision is more accurately called "denial."

So what does forgiveness look like?

No, really. When we summon the courage to look at it honestly, pragmatically—for real—what is forgiveness? Is it the healing of a cut? Emotional amnesia? Is it the fish that slips off the hook or the hungry fisherman left behind? Or is forgiveness the ability to see the good in someone even after they've harmed us?

Forgiveness does not require us to makes excuses for the person who wronged us or to forget that wrong was done; forgiveness requires us to believe that they are still capable of good, that they still have value, that they have good intentions and the ability to learn, even as we learn, from the devastating consequences of their mistake. Had Dr. Humano learned anything from his mistake? Did it make him a better surgeon? I hoped so, but I had no way to know other than to look him in the eye and ask him.

Before I could truly forgive Dr. Humano, I would have to confront him.

Seventeen

The holidays were a busy blur, as always, and I was careful about budgeting my energy, conserving my strength, and reserving the best of myself for my children. I'd done all my Christmas shopping online, which left a cluttered stack of cardboard boxes. In January, full of *new year/new you* resolve, I found breaking down those boxes one by one for recycling was a strangely meditative exercise.

I came upon Marie Kondo's book *The Life-Changing Magic of Tidying Up* and attacked my closet first. I purged years of designer handbags, suits and dresses I'd worn to satisfy someone else's image of me, restrictive foundation garments, uncomfortable shoes, and anything that didn't fit and flatter my altered body. I wasn't resigning myself to the idea that the shape of my body would never improve. I was simply accepting that this was the body I needed to live in at this moment. And every body, in every shape and every moment, deserves love.

This was about budgeting energy, choosing battles, and giving up control. High heels, tight clothing, bulky bags—these things were so not sparking joy for me. But maybe they could for someone else. I bagged the items that no longer belonged to me and folded the ones that did, exactly as the book instructed, so that the pants and sweaters looked like a neat library of color-coordinated books on a shelf. I liked the feeling of traveling light, an efficient tourist.

Next, I went to my grateful corner. Somehow, over the past two years, it had gone from a little moment of Zen to something that looked like a yard sale. Every item I touched meant something to me. Most were gifts that came directly from the heart of the giver—strange little figurines, embossed cards, ornate picture frames, and even a little bottle of chalky liquid that was supposed to be the breast milk of Mary, Mother of Jesus. A friend of Mami's had given it to me when I was trying to get pregnant, and in that moment, it had great meaning for me—not because I believed it was some magical holy relic but because it demonstrated the depth of her good heart. Every one of these items was a concentrated dose of loving energy that blessed me in the moment I received it. It was that moment that mattered, I realized. Hanging on to the items now was like trying to hold on to a kiss. You let go. The meaning and memory remain. (And you don't have to dust meaning and memory.)

I went through the bedroom closets with Lore and Paty, putting them to the task.

Holding up every frilly dress and pleated skirt, I asked, "Does this spark joy for you?"

"No."

Lore was decisive and emphatic about each item. Like me, she was surprised to discover the eye-opening power of that simple question.

"How about these?" I held up a pair of battered sneakers.

"Yes!"

The joy-sparking items that stayed in her closet were a random batch of skirts, jeans, T-shirts, and sandals that spoke volumes about what it means to be a happy, healthy kid.

It took me a few weeks, but I was on a mission to declutter, clarify, and spark joy in every closet and corner of my home—and somehow that extended to the closets and corners in my head. The traumatic events of the past year had left me shaken and sleepless. I knew the insomnia might be a reaction to one of the drugs I was taking, but I was taking so many different drugs, I didn't know which one I was reacting to. Symptoms came and went—heart palpitations, blood pressure spikes, mysterious rashes—necessitating a brain scan, biweekly lab work, and frequent visits to the doctor. In my wounded imagination, every headache was a brain tumor, every stomach bug a bleeding ulcer. If I developed a fever, I rushed to the ER. I longed for the restorative REM sleep I used to know. Napping doesn't cut it; the body needs deep, healing sleep.

Each doctor I saw—endocrinologist, OB/GYN, cardiologist, hematologist—saw me through the lens of their individual specialty. They saw the symptom. They didn't see *me*. I wanted their expert advice, and looking back, I see that I listened to them more than I listened to myself because I was still feeling skittish and fragile. The key to managing all this was balance, and I would have to find that balance within myself. I valued their professional opinions, but I was the only one with a full 360-degree view.

"The body has a higher wisdom," said Renu. "It will tell you what's needed."

I visited Renu every Tuesday, and she taught me about the healing power of colors, food, and meditation. We talked at length about the journey of the soul—the heroic journey—and how the endless circling of the universe sweeps humanity along. I liked talking about these things with someone whose belief system was so different from mine, someone who didn't require me to believe what she believed—or even to believe what *I* believed. I found it very liberating to say, "I don't know." I took in all the varied outlooks around me, free to apply what was useful, feeling no need to judge what might be useful for others.

Nonetheless, it was a lot to process—too much to process on my own. I got a referral to a good psychiatrist and drove downtown to meet with him one crisp, sunny morning in February.

Dr. Sidwell (not his real name) was a pleasant gentleman in his late fifties with thick eyebrows that matched his salt-and-pepper hair. His office made me feel like I was stepping into an old detective novel. The decor was a fusty mélange of accessible beige and faded Kelly green. I sat on one end of a disconcerting green sofa. He sat across from me in a loafer-brown side chair, a yellow legal pad balanced on his knee. Every once in a while he jotted something on the pad, taking notes without breaking eye contact, smiling and nodding as I told him about my family.

"So, what brings you here today?" he asked. "Tell me what's going on."

I told him the whole sordid tale, starting with my frustration over the delayed diagnosis, working up to the horrific plot twist. It really did sound like a telenovela. Dr. Sidwell's hedge of eyebrows came together in a tight furrow. He scribbled a few furious notes on the yellow pad and said, "Wait. Wait. You're saying he took out the wrong adrenal gland?"

"Yes."

"And this happened here in Austin?"

"Yes."

"Do you mind if I ask the surgeon's name?"

When I said Dr. Humano's name, the color drained from Dr. Sidwell's face.

"My daughter is scheduled for surgery with him next week," he said. "I should call her. She didn't want to wait, but . . . my God. I should tell her. Shouldn't I? Do you think I should call her?"

"Um . . . that's really not for me to say."

"Maybe she should reschedule. I mean, is he—I don't know. Do you think he's a good guy?"

"A good guy . . ."

I had no idea what this meant or how to answer, but I knew that I did not want to own this. *This*, I finally understood, this is why it made me so uncomfortable when people laid this at my feet when they were trying to push that lawsuit on me. "You don't want him to do this to someone else, do you?" As if that would be my fault. As if it were my responsibility every time he picked up a scalpel for the rest of his career. What if this experience actually made him a better surgeon? What if this young woman went to a different surgeon who hadn't recently received the wake-up call from hell and that surgeon made a careless mistake? Wouldn't that also be my burden to carry? If I took ownership of this, I was damned no matter what I did. Whether I decided to go through with this lawsuit or not, the decision had to be about me, not him.

It was time to make that decision. Almost two years had passed since the bungled surgery. There's a statute of limitations, the lawyer kept reminding me. I couldn't put it off much longer, and I didn't want to. I'd become very clear about what I needed. First, I needed to make peace with what happened, and in order to achieve that sense of closure, I would have to forgive Dr. Humano. Second, I needed to effect some small but meaningful change in a health care culture that functions as an incubator for disastrous outcomes. This wasn't about one doctor who botched one surgery. Patients are routinely ignored until we're in full-blown crisis mode. We're criticized, blamed, and eye-rolled. And then we're supposed to stuff our feelings and get back to normal. I couldn't go along with that anymore. If I felt any responsibility here at all—beyond accepting responsibility for my own body—it was to disrupt the old idea of *normal*.

Anyway . . .

Dr. Sidwell made an effort to collect himself and continue the appointment, but it was downhill from there. Distracted, he spoke about generic emotional responses to hypothetical trauma, hormones, statistics, blah blah blah, and then I left. I didn't make another appointment, but he called me a few days later to follow up. He seemed genuinely concerned, and I appreciated that, so I gave it another try, but the second appointment felt awkward, and I didn't go back.

"He did give me a prescription for sleeping pills," I told Renu. "That's something, I guess."

"What kind of sleeping pills?" Renu has very little use for Western medicine and was immediately suspicious.

"These."

I showed her the label, and she said, "Lorena, no. This is an antipsychotic. This is not something you take casually to help you sleep. And what about all the other medications you're taking? Did he ask about that? Because the interaction of these drugs could be dangerous."

He hadn't asked, and though I intended to do some research, I hadn't gotten that far yet. I was focused on a new issue with my pituitary gland malfunctioning, which the endocrinologist ultimately determined was because of the sleep aid. It never crossed my mind to ask him, "Say, will this drug have an adverse influence on my pituitary gland?" I depended on him to ask the right questions. He's the one who went to medical school! He knew what had happened to me and that I was on a variety of medications.

When I did dive into the research, I discovered that the Department of Justice and the Department of Health and Human Services had recently ordered a pharmaceutical giant to pay $520 million for illegally marketing this medication to psychiatrists for off-label uses, such as sleeplessness. Trust me, that was nothing to them. Pharmaceutical industry millions are like dog years. It's a whole different paradigm.

This massive lawsuit took place four years before Dr. Sidwell wrote that prescription for me. Five. Hundred. Million. Dollars. And the lawsuit had done exactly nothing to protect me. I was fooling myself to think that my little malpractice suit for a few hundred thousand was going to make any difference to anyone, and the thought of it going on for months or even years felt like the opposite of healing. We spent hours on speakerphone with the lawyers, and those conversations seemed to be taking me even further from my goal of forgiveness.

"I don't want to disappoint Eduardo," I confided in Renu, "but all this stress, all this effort and expense—I don't even know what it's for. It heals nothing. It teaches nothing. It changes nothing."

"Then do something else," said Renu. "Share what you've learned. Write a book."

I sat with this idea for a while, and it started to resonate. Writing a book would be a huge task, and I didn't know exactly how to go about it, but it fit with everything I learned from the example of my father and everything I was feeling in my heart of hearts. Being ignored had felt like a profound injustice. Maybe I'd find some sense of justice in making myself heard.

On a couples ski trip to Aspen that spring, I wanted to hide every time someone brought up the topic of the lawsuit. While everyone was chatting in front of the fire one evening, I slipped away and crawled into a bunk bed, huddling by a particular window where I was able to get a bar or two of cell phone signal. I knew in my heart I'd made the decision that was right for me, but I needed to check my compass. I called Papi and told him, "I don't want to disappoint you and Eduardo, but I'm not going through with the lawsuit. I want to forgive."

"That's very admirable, but he's never asked for your forgiveness. Never apologized. Never said another word to you about it."

This bothered me. A lot. Dr. Blevins, who was not the one at fault, had followed up with me, promptly answering texts and returning phone calls within a few hours, while Dr. Humano went radio silent. At the time, I needed to hear from him. Now I needed him to hear me.

Papi listened as I poured out my heart, finally articulating all these things that had been coming together in my head over two long years of confusion and misery, everything I'd come to understand about the broader definition of justice, meaningful change, and authentic forgiveness. I told him that I still intended to pursue those goals by writing a book and that I'd already decided not to use Dr. Humano's name—though the lawyer assured me that I could—because I didn't want my story to carry any whiff of side-eyed revenge.

When I stopped speaking, there was a long moment of thoughtful silence, in which I felt every part of me leaning in to hear Papi's answer. I didn't need his permission, but I valued his advice and hoped I might feel a spark of pride in his voice.

"That's why I have always loved you," he said. "Few people would have come to this conclusion." He sat with all this for another long moment, then took a deep breath in and let it out. "You have my support."

We talked for a while about the nuts and bolts of it all. All my life, I'd told my stories with art. I was unfamiliar with this work and with the world of publishing, but for him, it had always been his daily bread.

"The last piece of the story is still out there," I said. "I need to speak with Dr. Humano face-to-face."

My father offered some wise counsel about that meeting, and I kept his words at the front of my mind as I went forward with my plan.

"Prepare yourself," he said. "Send him a letter in advance. Make sure he knows that you are strong, that you've thought this through."

"*After giving it some deep thought . . .*" I teased, because that's how my father always started letters to me and my siblings. He'd go on to lay out the issue at hand, his feelings about it, and what he saw as a possible solution. He applied the same method to professional correspondence. His letters were carefully worded, dispassionate, and to the point. "I make it bulletproof," he always said. "Then I shoot."

"You're not asking him to guide you," said Papi. "You're expecting him to listen. He owes you that, to say the very least. Clarify your goals for the meeting—in your own mind and in the letter—so you both know why you're there."

"And when I get there . . ."

"When you get into that room, don't let go of the microphone. He'll try to explain himself or perhaps lay blame. He'll want to tell his story, and that is not the story you're there to discuss. You can't control the outcome. His response is his response. But you can control that meeting so he doesn't cause you any further harm."

I called Dr. Humano's office and set up the meeting, and then I wrote a clear, carefully worded letter, which I ran past my father before sending.

> *Dr. Humano:*
> *I write to you with the intention of creating and making positive experiences out of a very hard and unfortunate one.*
>
> *In truth, being left alone without guidance during such a hard process was very hurtful. There was a lot of*

stress and uncertainty in my life. But I need to admit that, through those heartbreaking months, I encountered some beautiful blessings.

I recently have learned to appreciate a concept I had previously not given much thought to: the law of unintended consequences.

There have been great benefits from the unexpected calamity of having the wrong adrenal gland removed.

At first, it was not easy for me to internalize the right attitude—one that would help me grow. There were too many moving parts, and I needed to stabilize my emergency health condition.

At first, it was a matter of survival.

Now, I have taken a different view.

I've learned that you must become your own advocate for your health.

I've learned that revenge is about inflicting harm on someone for a wrongdoing. And by having revenge in my mind, I was only detrimenting myself.

We learn from mistakes—our own, and those of others. I have embraced the positive view.

I am positive, because I want to learn about your process as a doctor and what you encountered.

I am positive, because I want to find answers for how we can work as a team to forge a trusting relationship between patients and doctors. How we can help doctors to not fear their own patients.

Perhaps unintended consequences can be the key to something much bigger.

I invite you to think about negative things that have turned out positive. A knowledge gained that might be of benefit.

Can we meet and talk without fear, anger, or reproach?
About something good learned out of turmoil.

Where mistakes transform into something bigger
than life.

Very best,
Lorena Junco

On the way to Dr. Humano's office, I felt calm and focused. I was prepared, and I was ready—and yes, there is a difference. Writing the letter had prepared me, and I was so ready, after all these months, to lay down this burdensome moment and move forward from it. I was ready to shed the heaviness of anger and grief. I was dressed in the sacred, healing colors of life—orange, yellow, and red—comfortable in my skin and steady on my feet.

Eduardo was nervous enough for both of us. He'd made it clear that he didn't trust or forgive Dr. Humano, and I had to respect that. Eduardo had made his own terrible journey during the past two years. There was no way I could fully understand it any more than he could fully understand mine. The best we could do was to respect each other's right to own and process the experience, each in our own way. Still, I had to admonish him about his place in the room.

"I know you still have a lot of anger," I said, "but this isn't about you or your anger. This is my moment to be heard. If you can't support that, I need you to wait for me outside."

"I just hope you're not expecting him to be changed by this," said Eduardo. "That would be a waste of energy."

"I have no expectations of anyone but myself," I assured him. I had to accept that Dr. Humano had the right and responsibility to process his experience in his own way as well. But I continued to quietly hope.

Eduardo promised to be cool, and I knew I could depend on that promise. I was glad to have him by my side. There was an uncomfortable moment when we first arrived; the receptionist had no idea who I was or why I was there, and Dr. Humano wasn't there. When he did arrive, striding his big lanky stride, he was wearing scrubs. It felt like we were being reminded that he was busy, going about the important business of life and death, and we were privileged to have a moment of his time.

As my father predicted, Dr. Humano was eager to steer the conversation with his own story. This was his first malpractice case, he assured me. Nothing—*nothing*—like this had ever happened, not in all his hundreds of surgeries.

"Then what happened?" I asked. "I need to know how you made this terrible mistake."

"I don't . . . I'm . . . I *always* look at the scans," he said.

"But you didn't look at mine." I nodded to the framed family pictures on his desk. "What would you have done differently if I were your daughter?"

Tears coursed down his cheeks. He started talking about how he had such and such credentials and did so many things pro bono, how he had saved so many lives and had nothing but the utmost concern for his patients.

"*I'm* your patient," I said, and he had no answer for that. (There's an old Spanish saying: "Be careful when you spit upward.")

I thought of my father's advice, maintaining control of the microphone, making sure the conversation was about me.

"Doctor, I'm not here to learn about your other patients. I'm here to tell you about the past two years of my life. About how I and my family suffered. How Dr. Blevins followed up with me, cared for me, and took ownership of this, even though it was not his mistake. I was heartbroken that I never heard a word from you. Not in all this time. I imagine you were following the advice of your lawyers.

My lawyers had strong advice for me, too. I chose for myself to do what I felt was right. We all choose for ourselves."

I went on to say what I needed to say, expanding only a little on what I'd written in the letter. Throughout the conversation, my voice was strong and even, while his voice sounded shaken to the core.

"I forgive you," I said, without waiting for him to say, "I'm sorry"—which he never really did. He said things like, "I'm sorry you had to go through this" or "I'm sorry that happened." If I'd waited for him to ask my forgiveness, I'd be waiting still. And that's okay. Because this was about me, not him.

He was enthusiastic when I offered to partner with him in an effort to improve communication on the part of patients and understanding on the part of doctors, nodding and agreeing as I spoke about how we might work together to effect meaningful, lasting change in surgical culture. We parted with promises to email and plans to follow up on my ideas.

"May I give you a hug?" I asked.

"Of course!"

He scrambled to his feet, obliging me with a brief but firm embrace. When I put my arms around him, I found the back of his shirt drenched in sweat.

I never saw him again.

eighteen

One evening when Eduardo and I were out for a drive, he seemed very pensive, so I asked him, "What are you thinking?"

"When I was a kid," he said, "I always dreamed of driving a sports car. I knew what the color would be. All the details. Then one day I had the opportunity to drive one. The exact car I dreamed of. And it didn't feel the way I thought I would feel."

"Because you've matured," I said.

The day we met with Dr. Humano, I left his office, holding Eduardo's hand, and I thought, *This conversation was my equivalent of the sports car.*

The meeting provided closure, but it didn't change anything. It didn't change me, and though I could never truly know, I doubted that it had changed Dr. Humano. Everything went exactly as I had hoped it would. Everything I needed to say, I said, and there was nothing I needed to hear. No part of my hopes or expectations hinged on any particular response from him. I didn't ask for an apology, and no apology was offered. He behaved exactly as he should have in this little vignette, but he seemed cautious, maybe even coached.

Years later, sorting all this out with a wonderful therapist (who reminds me of Mr. Rogers), I asked, "What if a doctor came to you and said, 'I hurt someone in a way that can never be made right.' How would you advise him?"

"First," said my therapist, "I would say, 'Good on you for taking ownership of it.' And then I would recommend a three-step apology. Step one: full ownership. 'I'm sorry I hurt you by taking your adrenal gland.' Step two: take it back—not in the sense of undoing it, but speaking to his own midbrain, saying, 'I take it back. I will never do that again.' And step three: find the lesson. Maybe multiple lessons. 'How did I let this happen? What did I do that facilitated this? I wish I had done XYZ instead.' And then, if the opportunity exists, I would tell him to offer reparations. 'What can I do to earn your forgiveness? Can I repair this with you?' It's the opposite of mea culpa."

I hope Dr. Humano has found equally wise counsel in his neighborhood. I hope he's found the strength to take ownership of what he did, because if he doesn't own it, he'll never truly forgive himself, but it's not my burden to make him better or make him stop. I was sincere when I invited him to join with me in an effort to improve doctor-patient communications, and that door will always be open, but I wasn't surprised when months and then a year and then another year went by in radio silence.

When I told my father about the meeting, I said, "Thank you for your advice. I took a lot of strength from it. I'm glad you were there with me in that way. You respected me enough to let me handle it myself instead of roaring in to stand up for me. I know that wasn't easy for you. Eduardo, too. He was strong. He managed himself very well."

"Did you tell the doctor you intend to write a book?" Papi asked.

"Yes," I said. "He was all for it. He wished me luck and said I should feel free to use his name."

My father smiled a knowing smile. "He does not believe for a moment that you will actually see it through—or that anyone will care if you do."

I had already assumed as much myself, but it was immaterial to me if Dr. Humano or anyone else believed I would, could, or should share my story in a book. I knew I would. And I knew that if I called him out by name, it would cast a fog of vengeance over what I really wanted to say: that it was forgiveness that changed me, not the surgery or the confrontation or the closure.

Forgiveness seemed so hard when I tried to pursue it on principle, a noble goal. When I stopped trying to force it, it happened. I opened the doors and windows of my soul, and forgiveness moved through me like fresh air.

I can't identify the exact moment. Maybe during that conversation with my father in Aspen when I finally found the courage to let go of the lawsuit. Or maybe when I read Renu the letter I wrote to Dr. Humano. Hearing the lines out loud, I felt every word come from my heart. I was trembling at the start and sobbing by the end, weak with relief, free from the vise grip of the whole bloody thing. My tears flowed, and it felt good. Renu always says I'm "very watery, very fluid"; I'm sure this is not what she had in mind.

"You are being called toward surrender," she said. "I know about this in theory, having studied and meditated on it in depth for twenty years and having helped a few clients on this journey. I have never done it fully myself. You are my teacher. You passed the ultimate test." Not long ago, Renu told me, "I remember falling to my knees after you left that day, thinking of my own journey—the journey of every soul, which ends, ideally, in freedom to live."

Years later, I am still humbled by those words.

Still learning. Still healing.

Still finding my way.

EPILOGUE

This is a love story because I chose to implement love as a lifestyle and adopt love as my homeland, but my forgiveness was for me—my peace of mind, my sense of self. Forgive does not mean forget. Forgetting would mean letting go of everything I've learned, and I'm not willing to do that. I say this with humble gratitude: forgiveness set me free, freedom allowed me to move forward, and moving forward, I was empowered to speak truth.

First, I had to speak truth to myself: *I'm angry.*

Second, I had to speak truth to Dr. Humano: *You wronged me.*

Now I hope to speak truth to you, my friend: *There is a way forward from anger and wrongdoing.*

My family and I have moved forward. Our life is good, even in those moments when we're forced to mourn a new loss or rework a persistent problem. The particulars are not suitable dinner conversation, and ultimately, those details aren't helpful, because everyone is different. What works or doesn't work for my body is not necessarily what works or doesn't work for your body. What is helpful, I hope, is knowing that even when my body fails me, I maintain a baseline happiness that makes this imperfect life worth living and this imperfect body worth loving.

My health issues are an issue. Instead of spending time on a tedious list of medications, restrictions, and long-term implications, let's close our eyes and think about the Gulf of Mexico. I'm sick of talking about how sick I can be. I've made peace with the reality of vigilant follow-up, blood work, medication, and occasional setbacks that will continue for the rest of my life. These things will always steer my schedule, but they will never define me.

People still ask me that loaded question: "How *are* you?" How I am is grateful. How I am is happy when happiness is available and hopeful when it is not. How I am is alive and determined to stay that way. How I am is a lot of things. There's no simple answer to that question, and that's fine. We're allowed to be whatever we need to be, and sometimes that means being more than one thing at the same time.

Last year, Eduardo and I studied for the US citizenship test. At night we'd lay down together and quiz each other. "How many amendments to the Constitution?" Supreme Court, history, politics—that was our pillow talk for a while. The day we passed the test, there was a mariachi band playing in the courthouse, and at home we celebrated with hot dogs, burgers, and apple pie. (Welcome to Texas!) We are now Mexican and *estadounidense*—citizens of the United States. People always say "American," but Mexicans are already American, remember. And maybe that's the metaphor. All the things you are, ultimately, are one thing: *you*. And that's a beautiful thing to be, if you can find your way there.

Eduardo found his own way to work out the rage and frustration. He never made that my responsibility. He was and is my protector, a man of few words who expresses his love for me with meaningful action. He throws himself into bold efforts and makes big things happen. He still plays soccer with the same joy he felt as a boy, kicking a ball down the field. He's not one to talk a lot about his feelings. He'd rather discuss the intricate engineering of a well-made motorcycle.

"It's like flying an airplane," says Eduardo. "You have to be fully engaged. On a motorcycle, you have to be there. You feel the flow of the road. You smell the field of corn. A good playlist is important. You need to keep the right music in your head."

I don't think he intends this to be a metaphor for living on the precious edge of life, but it's a good one.

"All the success and trouble makes you stronger," he says. "Extreme north and south. All you can do is hold on to the people around you."

Eduardo questioned my decision regarding the lawsuit, but he never questioned his faith in my ability to make that decision for myself. I have never regretted the decision I made, and this leaves some people shaking their heads. When I share the story of this tragic error as straightforwardly as I've shared it with you here, most people automatically assume that there was a lawsuit. They ask me quite bluntly: "How much did you get?" They assume some fantastic amount of money must result from such a clear-cut case of malpractice. The answer to that question is:

Nothing.

And everything.

Only a few people who went through it all with me understand that this tragedy—while it was not a gift in itself—opened my eyes to a host of hidden blessings. I'm not sure it's possible to truly know the great power of love and resilience within us until we're tested. It's the crucible moments in life, the refining fires, that strengthen and prove us, so forgiveness does not ask us to forget. It challenges us to forge a new self, capable of creating a new life. As I tell you my story, I hope you'll see something of your own story in it. I hope you'll look at your most challenging experiences and ask yourself, "How much did I get?" And if the answer is nothing—or worse than nothing—I hope you'll consider another point of view. Disaster does not happen in a vacuum. It happens in the context of a life, and life is rich with unseen gifts. Forgiveness is one of them.

Our children were so small when all this happened, we focused on the pretty side of forgiveness. They accepted this, along with the constant sales pitch of optimism. They were dented by the loss of me, but when they speak about that time—if they speak of it at all—it's as if I were living on another planet. There but not there. Alive but not living. The best I can do now is hold on to them and keep the right music in their heads.

As our children grow, Eduardo and I witness the far-reaching effects of what they went through. They're aware of my body, always wanting to be near me but careful about hugging me too hard. They've grown up with dinner conversations that covered the mechanics of humanity and the boundless possibilities of spirituality.

When Eduardo and I began planning the construction of Casa Lotus, Lore, Paty, and Eddie Jr. were old enough to appreciate the symbolism and aesthetics that steered the design, materials, and process. They had witnessed the power of destruction. I wanted them to see how reconstruction goes inward. The dream of Casa Lotus began as a spark within our broken hearts. I cleared the land for it when I forgave myself. I built the foundation as I regained my strength. We included them in the process from the beginning, talking with them about what this home would mean to our family and to each of them individually.

The day we broke ground at Casa Lotus and began the great artistic endeavor that will eventually be our home, we invited the architects and builder to join our family—including the members of our staff who have become family to us—in a ceremonial blessing of the site. Swami Shivatmananda performed the ceremony in

Hindi, so none of us understood a word of it, but we cried anyway. There was a meaning that transcended language and spoke to our souls. I felt the masculine and feminine energy embodied by Jesus and Mary, understanding that the moment meant something different to each of us.

Swami Ji offered a gift of fruit rinds and gold coins to Mother Earth and asked her to forgive this disruption to the land, the disturbance to the plants, ants, birds, and squirrels. Then he strode around the property for two hours with Lore, Paty, and Eddie following along behind him like ducklings. They were committed!

I see compassion in my children that you don't see in most people until much later in life, and I try to nurture that. Last summer, a young mother and her baby boy traveled to Texas from the Philippines so he could have heart surgery. Through HeartGift Foundation, an organization that provides lifesaving heart surgery to children from all over the world, we sponsored the surgery and hosted Mama and Baby in our home. In a thousand ways—practical, creative, and spilling over with love—Lore and Paty and even little Eddie participated in the extraordinary level of care this baby needed in the months before and after the delicate procedure. Their gentleness and empathy, their tenderness toward this child who was so little and needed so much—it brought tears to my eyes. I thought I was gifting this baby, but I understand now he gave me the gift of believing in the lifesaving powers of a doctor. I don't know what the future holds for my children, but I know they're brave enough to see it, strong enough to go there, and kind enough to bring one another along.

Compassion is a mind-set. Caregiving is a skill set. Both must be taught. They don't just happen. The heart is a muscle, remember? It grows larger when more is asked of it. The human body is capable of learning new tricks and work-arounds, I have learned. So is the soul.

About three years after the botched surgery, one of the other moms at school confided in me that she'd been feeling low. The symptoms she described were hauntingly familiar.

"Maybe you should ask them to check your adrenal glands," I said.

I didn't see her again for several months, but she and her family traveled a lot, so it wasn't unusual for her to be out of circulation for a while. One day at school, I spotted her in the auditorium just before the regular morning announcements. She was moving carefully. I could tell she was hurting and asked, "Are you okay?"

"I just had surgery," she said. "I'll tell you later."

"How can I help?"

She asked me to help her pull up a chair so she could sit. After announcements, I showed her where to find the elevator. (I know all the energy-conserving shortcuts.) We found a quiet moment to catch up before we went to our kids' classrooms. She told me she'd recently had surgery and that an amazing doctor had saved her life. He was humble and compassionate, she said. He asked questions and listened to the answers. He was diligent before and followed up after, making sure her recovery was on track. I felt a sting of envy, but I was glad to hear she'd found someone so caring, a surgeon who seemed to see the procedure in the context of her life. Then she mentioned the surgeon's name. It was Dr. Humano.

A wave of mixed emotions took my breath away. I had no words. This was not the time to pepper her with questions or unpack the story of my experience. That was a conversation for another day, but I knew I'd eventually have to tell her after she'd had a chance to regain her balance. It would feel weird not to. Meanwhile, I'd have to rein in any impulse to read a lot into it. Like the meeting with Dr. Humano, her story offered a modicum of closure, but it didn't really change anything.

I was glad for them both that it went well. It's not useful for me to spend time wondering why her experience with him was so different from mine, if he truly had changed, or if my experience had anything to do with who he is now. The stages of accountability are similar to the stages of grief: denial, anger, depression, bargaining, acceptance. Each one demands due diligence. From my perspective, I see that grief, accountability, and healing are intertwined. So, perhaps a sixth and final stage should be added to the customary algorithm: *forgiveness.*

Forgiveness is nothing more and nothing less than a way forward for the forgiver. The forgiven must find his own way. I had plenty of reasons to be skeptical about Dr. Humano's willingness to grow as a surgeon and human being. My only reason for hope is that I am a hopeful person, and an optimist is like a prickly pear: it is good at protecting itself, courageously survives long periods of neglect, and occasionally yields a vibrant blossom.

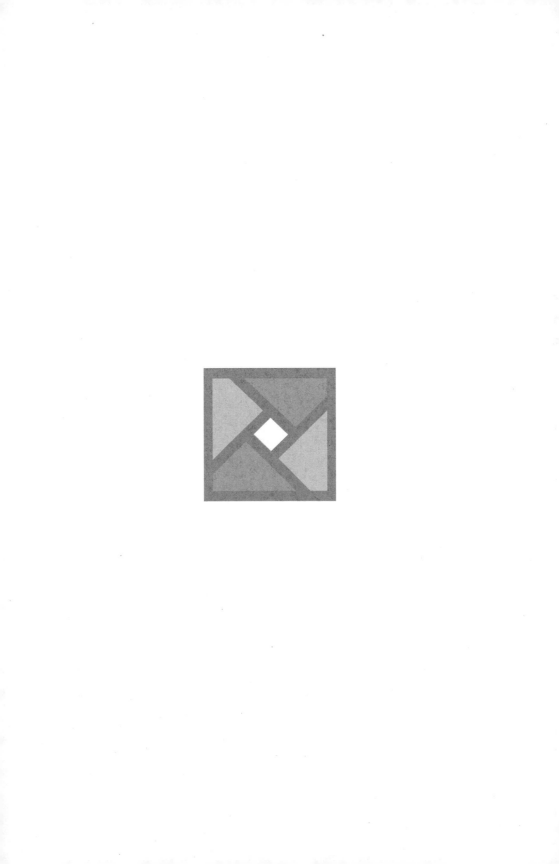

ACKNOWLEDGMENTS

It's impossible to fully express my deep, heartfelt gratitude:

To Eduardo, my husband, and our three treasures, Lore, Paty, and Eddie, who make me want to get up every morning.

To Mom and Dad and Tía Paty and Tío Ricardo, and all my close family for their unfailing love and support.

To my dearest "little" sister Roby, who has taught me nothing little. Her courage, boldness, and heart were my inspiration to fight for life.

To our personal staff, especially Blanca, for care and strength, and to all the medical staff who've taken such great care of me.

To Renu Namjoshi, my friend, counselor, and moral compass.

To Joni Rodgers for interpreting my thoughts as if we'd been friends since forever.

To all my friends, for their invaluable support and gestures of love.

Everyone has their own Casa Lotus, that place in your heart that brings out the ever-evolving best version of you. Whether you realize it or not, you are already on your way. To help reveal your road map, visit LorenaJuncoMargain.com to access resources and videos to support you in your journey.

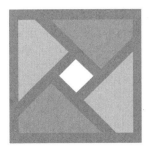

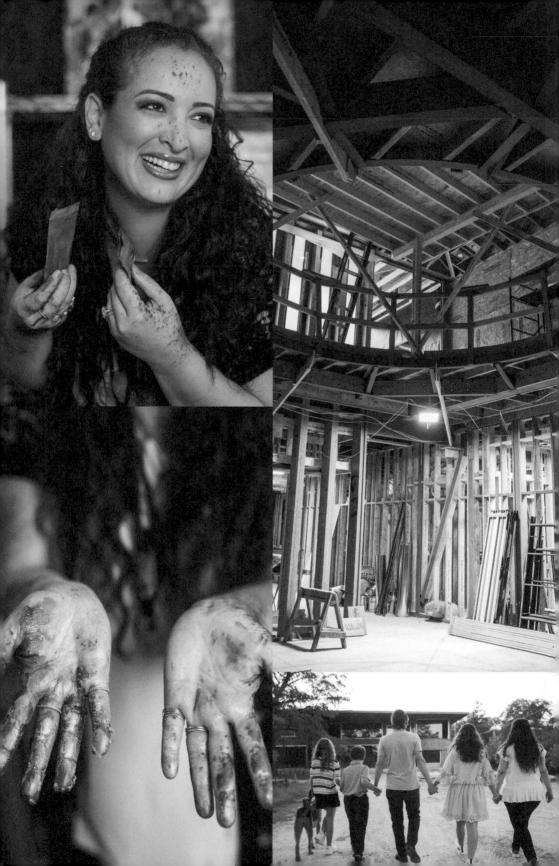